Get
Control
of Your
BLOOD
SUGAR

Gary Scheiner, M.S., C.D.E.

Publications International, Ltd.

Gary Scheiner, M.S., C.D.E., is a certified diabetes educator and exercise physiologist who has successfully managed his own diabetes since 1985. He has received several awards for his diabetes teaching, and he delivers lectures worldwide for patients and health care professionals. His private practice, Integrated Diabetes Services, features a team of diabetes educators specializing in healthy lifestyles and intensive blood sugar control. Consultations are available via phone and Internet; you can call toll-free 1-877-735-3648 or visit www.integrateddiabetes.com for more information.

Illustrations: Wendy Beth Jackelow, M.F.A., C.M.I.

Contents

Easy (Really) Does It!

RECENTLY, TWO NEW patients came to my office for diabetes counseling. Both were middle-aged men who, I think, were only there because their wives dragged them.

The first man had been living with type 2 diabetes for many years. He was on several diabetes medications, but his blood sugar levels had crept above normal again. "I don't get it," he said. "I do everything I'm supposed to do. I exercise every day. I watch what I eat. I even lost about 20 pounds. I test my blood twice a day. Every couple of years they add another medication; it works for a while, then my blood sugars start to go up again, and it seems like I'm back where I started. What gives?"

I asked him how he feels now compared to when he was diagnosed. A smile crept across his face, and he and his wife exchanged glances.

"No comparison. My clothes fit again, I've got more energy, and I can walk for more than an hour without getting tired. Things in the bedroom are better, too." His wife couldn't stop nodding.

After explaining to him that diabetes is a progressive disease that requires more aggressive treatment as time goes on, I congratulated him.

"What for?" he asked. "I know you're about to tell me I need to take another pill or start insulin. So why congratulate me?"

"You took something potentially negative and harmful and turned it into something positive and productive," I said. "For that, you deserve a lot of credit."

The second man had not been given an "official" diagnosis of diabetes by his physician, but he had been told years ago that his sugar level was up and he'd better make some changes. He didn't. By the time he came to my office, he was grossly out of shape: He had a huge potbelly and was unable to walk across the room without a great deal of effort. The fact that he breathed heavy during our conversation told me all I needed to know about the state of his cardiovascular system.

"He hasn't had a good night's sleep in months," his wife declared. "You're getting up what, five, six times a night?" He just nodded.

"I don't think he'd have come here today if the eye doctor hadn't found something wrong," she said. "He doesn't seem as sharp as he used to be, either. I think he needs to start taking the diabetes more seriously. I don't think he cares about it at all."

But the lines on his face told a different story. Here sat a man riddled with worry and guilt over an illness he just didn't think he could do much about.

"What's the point? If I've got it, I've got it. It's not like I can change it. All the testing and dieting and pills are too much for a guy my age. I might as well enjoy myself."

But this did *not* look like a man who was enjoying himself.

The differing paths of these two men reminded me of some sage advice my dad once gave me:

"There is an easy way and a hard way to do anything, so look for the easy way."

Dad probably meant something along the lines of "work smarter, not harder." But as an exercise physiologist and certified diabetes educator who counsels people with diabetes every day, and as a person with diabetes myself, I have come to realize that his advice takes on a whole new meaning when applied to living with type 2 diabetes. Sometimes, the "easy" way is really not so easy, and the "hard" way actually makes life easier.

The first man took the "hard road" to managing diabetes, but it wasn't all that complicated. He worked at it. He made some sacrifices and compromises along the way. He adapted to challenges as they arose. As a result, his life is really much easier now. He can do the things he likes to do without too much effort, and he enjoys himself. The "work" he's been putting into managing his blood sugar and taking care of his diabetes has become so much a part of his lifestyle, he doesn't even think of it as work.

He is proud of the positive changes he has made, and you can bet that he sleeps well at night.

The second man took the so-called "easy road" to managing diabetes. He ignored it. He ate all he wanted and didn't bother with pills or blood sugar tests. He likely chose TV over physical activity every chance he could. As a result, everything comes hard to him now—sleeping, seeing, breathing, the simple act of moving. My guess is he gets little true enjoyment from the abundant food and relaxation that have become staples of his life.

This book is all about helping you discover the ease with which type 2 diabetes can be managed, and how much easier life can be if you follow a set of simple steps to get and keep your blood sugar under control. If you'd prefer to take the truly "hard road" and avoid dealing with diabetes, this book is not for you. But if you're ready for a change in the way you view and manage your blood sugar problems, WELCOME ABOARD!

STEP 1:
Know Your Opponent

Understanding the ins and outs of diabetes will allow you to manage it more effectively.

BACK IN MY COLLEGE days, I was a pretty good poker player. Anyone who thinks winning at poker is simply a matter of luck knows nothing about the game. Sure, it helps if you're dealt decent cards, but it's more important to know the other players.

My buddy Craig, for example, would never bluff. It didn't matter what the situation was. If he didn't have a guaranteed winning hand, he would fold right away. Jeff was more of a "streak" player. If he lost a few hands in a row, he had a tendency to overbid in an attempt to win it all back at once. The other Jeff didn't know the game that well. Any time he had a wild card, he would bet big—even if he only had a pair. Bob was tougher to figure out because he knew how to play and liked to bluff sometimes. Luckily, he had a "tell." A tell is a quirky behavior that someone exhibits when they have a certain type of hand (good or bad). We always had tons of snacks on hand when we played, and Bob would start to eat faster than usual when he had a really good hand. So whenever Bob started plowing through the chips, I knew it was time to fold.

It also helped to know who was hard up for cash, because that player would tend to bet more conservatively. He would be easier to "buy out" with a large bet. And everyone knows that "unlucky at love" equals "lucky at cards." So if someone was on the outs with his girlfriend, I knew to watch out. That guy would be sure to clean up at the poker table.

Why the tutorial on the subtleties of low-stakes poker? Simple. In managing diabetes, just as in playing poker, knowing your opponent makes it easier to succeed.

Easy Diabetes Control Secret #1:
Knowing your opponent makes it easier to succeed.

And that's why this first step in your blood-sugar-control program is all about helping you to get to know your disease. Here we explain, in easy-to-understand terms, exactly what diabetes is. We uncover the underlying causes of the two main types of diabetes—who tends to get each, and why. And along the way, we reveal many of the factors in everyday life that affect blood sugar levels so that you gain a sense of what you're up against and what it's going to take for you to manage your blood sugar properly.

Let's get started!

What Type Are You?

Diabetes, in the simplest terms, refers to the body's inability to control blood sugar levels. Most of the food we eat is broken down by the body into a simple sugar called **glucose.** The glucose derived from our food is absorbed into the bloodstream and carried to all parts of the body so that it can be used for energy. **Carbohydrates** (sugars and starches) raise the blood sugar particularly quickly, but protein and fat can also increase blood sugar levels.

It is important to keep blood sugar levels within a certain range so that the body functions properly. If the blood sugar level drops too low, the body's cells become starved for energy. If it rises too high—and especially if it stays high—blood vessels become clogged and damaged, and body chemistry as a whole gets a bit out of whack.

Think of it this way: If you are making lemonade and put in too little sugar, the lemonade is going to taste bland and sour. Put in too much sugar, and it will taste disgustingly sweet. Having just the right *concentration* of sugar is essential for making the lemonade taste just right.

Insulin is very important to the whole process of blood sugar control. Insulin is a **hormone**, a special protein that has a special job to do. Once sugar enters the bloodstream, insulin is responsible for pulling it out of the blood and packing it into our body's cells. Get it? *Insulin* moves sugar *into* cells.

Insulin is made by the pancreas, an organ just below the stomach. The pancreas constantly measures blood sugar levels and produces just enough insulin to keep the blood sugar level within a normal range (approximately 70 to 110 milligrams per deciliter, or mg/dl, before meals). As blood sugar levels go up, especially after meals, the pancreas makes more insulin. As blood sugar levels drop between meals and when we are physically active, the pancreas makes less insulin.

Diabetes can be caused by two completely different problems. Either the pancreas does not produce enough insulin, or the insulin that is produced just doesn't work very well.

In someone with **type 1 diabetes,** the pancreas no longer makes any insulin at all. The part of the pancreas that produces insulin has been destroyed, accidentally, by the body's own immune system. That's why type 1 diabetes is called an **autoimmune disease.** The immune system is supposed to attack things like bacteria and viruses that don't belong in the body. It is supposed to recognize the various parts of its own body and leave them alone. In some people, however, the immune system does a poor job of recognizing the "good guys" (the body's own parts) and may attack them when hunting for the "bad guys" (foreign invaders) — sort of like firing bullets randomly into a big crowd of people that happens to contain a few villains. Since the pancreas is the only part of the body that can produce insulin, an autoimmune attack on the organ leaves the body without this essential hormone.

With no insulin available, most of the body's cells are unable to get the sugar they need to survive, even though there is a great deal of it floating around in the bloodstream. People with type 1 diabetes require insulin injections to control their blood sugar levels and stay alive. Type 1 diabetes is usually diagnosed during childhood or adolescence, but it can also appear for the first time in early adulthood.

The 3 Stages of Type 2 Diabetes

Stage 1: Insulin resistance

Stage 2: Failure to make enough insulin

Stage 3: Loss of pancreatic function

More than 90 percent of people with diabetes have what's called **type 2 diabetes.** Type 2 is very different from type 1 in that there is no autoimmune attack, and the pancreas continues to produce insulin. In fact, the pancreas may actually produce *more* insulin than it does in a person without diabetes.

Confused yet? Don't worry. Let's take a step back and look at what is really behind the development of type 2 diabetes.

Stage 1: The Resistance

In order to do its job of taking sugar out of the bloodstream and loading it into the body's cells, insulin attaches to something called a receptor on the outer surface of the cell. This is similar to the way a key enters a lock in order to open a door. Once insulin attaches to the receptor, a series of reactions takes place that allows the big sugar molecules into the cell.

For insulin to perform its job, therefore, there have to be sufficient receptors on the cell surface, and the chemical reactions inside the cell have to take place. When there are problems with the receptors or with the chemical reactions, we refer to this condition as **insulin resistance.** When the body's cells are insulin resistant, insulin becomes less effective at lowering the level of sugar in the blood.

What causes insulin resistance? Typically, it is a combination of genetics (heredity) and lifestyle. Family history plays a major role. Having close relatives with type 2 diabetes greatly increases your risk of the disease. Certain ethnic groups, including Native Americans, African Americans, Hispanic Americans, Asian Americans, and Pacific Islanders are also at high risk. The aging process plays a role as well. The older we get, the more insulin resistant we tend to become, so the risk of developing type 2 diabetes increases with age.

Killer Crossover?

People with type 1 diabetes can also develop type 2 diabetes later in life. Insulin resistance can develop in anyone who gains weight and has a genetic susceptibility to type 2 diabetes. But people with type 2 are very unlikely to develop type 1, even if they require insulin to control their blood sugar levels. They are referred to, simply, as **insulin-requiring type 2's.** True type 1 diabetes is caused by an immune system attack on the pancreas, not insulin resistance.

Women who have **polycystic ovary syndrome (PCOS)** often become insulin resistant due to the overproduction of certain hormones that work against insulin's action. Likewise, several hormones produced during pregnancy oppose insulin's action and can cause insulin resistance. **Gestational diabetes** is a form of type 2 diabetes that develops during and usually goes away at the end of pregnancy. However, women who have had gestational diabetes or have given birth to a large or heavy baby are at increased risk of developing type 2 diabetes as they get older.

Stressful circumstances, such as illness, injury, surgery, or daily emotional turmoil, also can cause significant insulin resistance. This is due to the production of stress hormones. These hormones normally prompt the surge of energy needed for a "fight or flight" response in stressful situations. Unfortunately for people prone to diabetes, the stress hormones trigger this energy burst by stimulating the liver to release extra sugar into the bloodstream and by causing insulin resistance.

A number of medications can also produce insulin resistance: most notably, anti-inflammatory steroid drugs such as cortisone and prednisone as well as certain medications that are used to treat asthma. These types of drugs create a state of insulin resistance throughout the body.

A lack of physical activity can cause insulin resistance in many people. The muscles are one of the primary consumers of sugar for energy. When muscle function is limited to little more than getting up to find the remote control or to head to the fridge, muscles start to lose their sensitivity to insulin. Even in people who are usually very active, a couple of days without much activity will result in some degree of insulin resistance.

Last but certainly not least, insulin resistance increases with body size. But let's get the terminology straight. We're not talking about being big and muscular. We're talking about having too much body fat, particularly around the midsection. Obesity (being more than 20 percent over one's ideal weight due to excess body fat) is far and away the number one risk factor for type

2 diabetes. We don't know exactly how body fat gets in the way of insulin. But we do know that fat cells secrete a hormone that limits insulin's ability to promote sugar uptake by the body's cells. The larger your fat cells, the more of this hormone you produce, and the greater your degree of insulin resistance. In fact, gaining as little as ten pounds over a 15-year period can double your level of insulin resistance.

Currently, more than 44 million Americans are considered to be obese. Compared to adults who weigh a healthy amount, obese individuals are more than *seven times* as likely to develop diabetes. And the problem is not restricted to adults: More than ever before, overweight children and teenagers are developing insulin resistance and type 2 diabetes. Each year, more than 5,000 American children ages 10 to 19 are diagnosed with type 2 diabetes, and the number is growing rapidly.

Stage 2: The Production Shortfall

Insulin resistance affects an estimated 60 to 75 *million* Americans. Why, then, do only some people with insulin resistance develop type 2 diabetes? Sure, the number of people with type 2 diabetes is growing at a pretty fast pace (5 percent per year), but currently only about 20 million Americans have been diagnosed with the disease. So why the discrepancy?

The reason is this: When insulin resistance occurs, the pancreas needs to produce more insulin to keep blood sugar levels in a normal range. In most cases, the pancreas can produce enough extra insulin to keep blood sugar levels in a normal range, even though the insulin is not working as well as it should. This is called the **pre-diabetes** phase.

But not everyone's pancreas has this capacity.

A Rose by Any Other Name...

If you've been diagnosed with **pre-diabetes,** take it every bit as seriously as you would the full-fledged disease. Pre-diabetes means that you are already insulin resistant and that your pancreas is beginning to show signs of wear. You can bet your bottom dollar that, if you don't make some important lifestyle changes, your condition will progress to a more severe state. So attack diabetes early—before your pancreas loses its capabilities and resilience.

Each person's pancreas can only crank up insulin production so much. Once the degree of insulin resistance is too much for the pancreas to overcome, blood sugar levels are going to rise above normal. In other words, a body must have both insulin resistance *and* a limit to its pancreas' ability to secrete extra insulin in order for elevated blood sugars—and type 2 diabetes—to occur.

To understand this concept better, imagine that you are an air conditioner trying to keep the house cool on a hot summer day.

If you're one of those high-powered central air-conditioning units that can crank out a bazillion BTUs, you'll have no problem overcoming the heat and keeping the house cool. But if you're one of those inexpensive window units, you're probably not going to be able to blow enough cold air to keep the entire house cool on a really hot, humid day.

In this example, the heat and humidity are like insulin resistance: They present a challenge to our comfort and well-being. The air conditioner is like the pancreas: An efficient system can overcome any challenge, but a less-resilient system can't. When a sluggish pancreas combines with major insulin resistance, the result is going to be type 2 diabetes.

At this early stage of type 2 diabetes, blood sugar control can often be achieved through exercise and a healthy diet. Physical activity, as we will discuss in a later step, helps the body overcome insulin resistance. Consuming fewer carbohydrates helps to limit the amount of sugar entering the bloodstream at any one time. And the combination of exercise and reduced food intake produces weight loss, which also improves insulin sensitivity. Sometimes at this stage, however, oral medications may also be needed to help the pancreas (or to help insulin) work more effectively. Combined with the lifestyle adjustments, they may be sufficient to rein in blood sugar levels. But in most cases, they won't be enough for long.

Stage 3: The Snowball Effect

Type 2 diabetes is a progressive illness. The word *progressive* in this context does *not* mean something positive. There is nothing hip, cool, or modern about it. In this case, *progressive* means that the disease will grow worse and become harder to control over time. When diabetes has been present for a number of years, insulin resistance tends to grow worse, and the pancreas struggles to keep up with the huge demand for insulin. Then a new problem typically sets in. Just like an air conditioner that is forced to run full blast every minute of every day, the pancreas starts to break down. (Heck, if you were asked to work day after day without any breaks and with no end in sight, you would break down too . . . or at least find a new job!)

The breakdown of the pancreas has two causes: Overwork and a condition known as **glucose toxicity.** The overwork part, we can all understand: Force those poor little pancreatic cells into relentless slave labor, and many of them are going to bite the dust. Glucose toxicity is a bit more complex.

Glucose, which is another word for the sugar we've been talking about, is a good thing in the right amounts. But as the saying goes, even too much of a good thing can be harmful. Elevations in blood sugar levels can actually damage the pancreas, further reducing its ability to produce insulin. So over time, as a result of the constant battle against insulin resistance, the pancreas starts to make less and less insulin.

This is why the treatment for type 2 diabetes usually must become more aggressive over time. It is why 40 percent of the people with type 2 diabetes take insulin injections, sometimes several times each day. Does this mean they now have type 1 diabetes? No, it does not. Remember, the type of diabetes is defined by what *caused* it, not how it is treated. Type 1 diabetes occurs when the body's own immune system destroys the part of the pancreas that makes insulin. Type 2 diabetes is caused by insulin resistance (usually due to obesity and family history/ ethnicity), followed by insufficient insulin production (as the pancreas fails to keep up with the increased demand), followed by a gradual breakdown of the pancreas (due to constant over-work and glucose toxicity).

Going back to one of our original statements, one thing that all forms of diabetes have in common is an inability to properly regulate blood sugar levels. Now that you know exactly what causes type 2 diabetes, the next step is to learn and remember why it is so vitally important to keep those blood sugar levels under control.

STEP 2:
Focus on Control's Immediate Benefits

Understanding the improvements you'll experience right away can provide powerful motivation to start reining in your runaway blood sugar.

B EING A PARENT has taught me a lot, especially about the value of responsibility and sacrifice. I've seen each of my four kids through their share of illnesses and injuries over the years. But none had a greater effect on me than when my youngest daughter was five years old and had a really bad case of the flu. She was vomiting a lot and became so dehydrated and feverish that we had to take her to the emergency room. They perked her up a bit by giving her intravenous fluids, but she was still really miserable. And she seemed so little and defenseless against that virus.

My wife and I weren't sleeping much through that ordeal. My wife did not catch the flu, but she did develop a nasty cold, probably because her immune system was so strained from all the stress. After we left the hospital, I tried to go to the office to see a few patients and catch up on messages, but I just wasn't myself.

I couldn't focus on other people's blood sugar levels when my mind was so wrapped up with my daughter's situation. I remember trying to go for a run to clear my head. I usually run three or four times a week, but I hadn't had a good workout since she got sick. I made it halfway down the block and had to stop. I just felt physically and emotionally drained, like my heart just didn't have anything left to give.

Thankfully, my daughter recovered from that illness soon enough and had no lasting negative effects from it. What surprised me most about the whole episode wasn't the effect it had on her, but the effect it had on me and my wife. *Our* inability to function under those circumstances taught me something important: Everything comes easier when you're free to focus.

Our bodies and our minds perform much better when we're not weighed down with burdens that are too large or too numerous. From a diabetes standpoint, having uncontrolled blood sugar is like going about your day with a huge, heavy yoke around your neck. That cumbersome yoke makes it much harder for you to do the things you want to do, accomplish all that you need to accomplish, and live each day to the fullest. On the other hand, lifting the yoke of runaway blood sugar levels frees you to focus on getting the most from each day. Every task becomes easier, and your life as a whole improves immediately when your blood sugar is well controlled.

That may sound like a bit of an exaggeration, but it is not. When you learn how many of your body's basic and advanced functions are affected by out-of-control blood sugar, and when you discover that regaining control can improve them right away, you'll realize just how much you stand to gain by getting your blood sugar levels in line.

Easy Diabetes Control Secret #2:

Everything else in life comes easier when uncontrolled blood sugar isn't interfering with your focus.

Step 3 discusses the long-term effects of diabetes—and the long-term benefits of improved blood sugar control. But what really tends to motivate most people is *immediate gratification*. What will you give me for my efforts *right now?* I'm not talking next month or next year or ten years down the road. I mean *right now!* So here in Step 2, we discuss some of the ways that you will be rewarded immediately for getting your blood sugar levels under control, including:

- Increased energy
- More restful sleep
- Improved physical performance
- Decreased appetite

- Heightened brain power

- More stable moods and emotions

- Fewer sick days

- Softer skin and healthier gums

- Greater personal safety

Focusing on the many impressive benefits you'll experience right away can provide you with powerful motivation to start managing your diabetes today.

Increased Energy

Raise your hand if you like being tired all the time. Okay, raise your hand if you're too tired to raise your hand. Elevated blood sugar reduces your overall energy level. Remember, high blood sugar is a sign that not enough sugar is getting into your body's cells, where it is used for energy. The fuel is there; it's just stuck in the bloodstream, kind of like a fleet of gasoline trucks that drive around aimlessly instead of unloading at your local gas station. This shortage of fuel inside the body's cells causes sleepiness and sluggishness. Even if the blood sugar is only elevated temporarily, the lack of energy will be noticeable during that time. As soon as the blood sugar returns to normal, the energy level usually improves. So forget the gimmicky "energy drinks." If you want more energy, control your diabetes!

More Restful Sleep

We all know how important a good night's sleep is to feeling well and being productive the following day. Unfortunately, diabetes makes you more prone to developing sleep disorders, including sleep apnea, a potentially life-threatening disorder in which the sleeper snores loudly and actually stops breathing multiple times throughout the night. Poor blood sugar control also reduces the *quality* of your sleep. If you've ever woken up from a really long night's sleep feeling as though you hardly got any rest at all, it may be because you never reached a deep phase of sleep. Having elevated blood sugar during the night keeps you at a shallow sleep level and prevents you from entering the deep, restful sleep you really need.

If your blood sugar is high enough, you might even wake up several times during the night to run to the bathroom. This is caused by a condition called **urine diuresis.** When blood sugar reaches more than twice the normal level, some of the sugar spills into the urine—and it drags a lot of water along with it. As the bladder fills, it wakes you up. The result may be frequent nighttime urination and even bedwetting. If the thought of a restful, uninterrupted, "dry" night's sleep appeals to you, control your diabetes!

Decreased Appetite

It might sound totally backward, but high blood sugar levels tend to make you crave more food—especially carbohydrate-rich food. Remember, it's not the amount of sugar in the bloodstream that counts, it's how much of that sugar gets into the body's cells. If not enough is getting into the cells, particularly the cells that regulate appetite, the body is going to feel hungry. Given that weight control is so important to both diabetes management and to your long-term health, it makes all the sense in the world to control your diabetes as well as possible.

Improved Physical Performance

Elevated blood sugar can reduce your strength, flexibility, speed, and stamina. So whether you're an aspiring athlete or just hoping to make it up a flight of stairs, you can immediately boost your physical abilities by gaining control of your blood sugar.

Muscles prefer sugar as fuel for making quick, intense movements. When the sugar in the bloodstream can't get into the muscle cells, therefore, strength suffers. Extra sugar in the bloodstream also leads to something called **glycosylation** of connective tissues, in which sugar coats tendons and ligaments, limiting their ability to stretch properly. Muscle stiffness, strains, and pulls are common in people with high blood sugar levels. High blood sugar also gunks up the connections between muscles and nerves, resulting in dulled reflexes and slower reaction times.

And extra sugar in the bloodstream limits the ability of red blood cells to pick up oxygen in the lungs and transport it to working muscles, causing rapid fatigue and restricted cardiovas-cular/aerobic capacity. So if you want to be able to perform well physically—during sports, exercise, or simple everyday activities—control your diabetes!

Trumping Diabetes with Tight Control

U.S. Olympic swimmer Gary Hall Jr. was diagnosed with diabetes in 1999. At the time of his diagnosis, he had competed for, but had never won, an individual gold medal. Even his doctors doubted that he would ever win a coveted individual gold after he developed diabetes. But through an intensive insulin program that helped him achieve very tight blood sugar control, Gary proved everyone wrong, capturing the individual gold in the 50-meter freestyle at the 2000 Olympics and again at the 2004 Games.

Heightened Brain Power

Blood sugar levels influence more than your muscles, ligaments, and tendons, however. Even your brain is affected. High blood sugar limits your ability to focus, remember, perform complex tasks, and be creative. Studies have repeatedly and consistently shown how mental performance suffers during periods of high blood sugar. As blood sugar goes up, so do mental errors and the time it takes to perform basic tasks. Wide variations in blood sugar levels, from early-morning lows to post-meal spikes, have also been shown to hinder intellectual function. If you (or your loved ones) have noticed a decline in your mental abilities, tightening control of your diabetes might be the answer. Likewise, if you want to perform as well as you possibly can at work, in school, or in a friendly game of bridge, keep an eye on those blood sugar levels.

Time for a New Career

Diabetes mellitus, the disease's full scientific name, is actually Latin for "urine like honey." The fact that people with diabetes have high levels of sugar in their urine has been recognized for thousands of years. The ancient Greeks used to describe diabetes as a mysterious illness that involved the melting down of flesh and limbs into urine. In A.D. 300, Indian and Chinese scholars observed that the urine of people with diabetes was remarkably sweet. Indeed, in ancient times, diabetes was commonly diagnosed by "water tasters" who sampled the urine (referred to back then as "water") of those suspected of having diabetes in order to detect the telltale sweetness. Luckily for the water tasters, another method of sugar detection soon replaced this practice: The urine was poured near an anthill instead. If the ants were attracted to the urine, it meant that the urine contained high levels of sugar.

More Stable Moods & Emotions

Besides intellectual performance, your brain is also responsible for maintaining your emotional balance. The fact is, your moods change along with your blood sugar level. (If you don't believe me, ask your partner!) High blood sugar levels can make you impatient, irritable, and generally negative. Achieving normal blood sugar levels *and keeping them there* can go a long way toward improving your mood and your emotional stability. That's not to say that you will become an instant optimist or the life of the party, but the way you interact with your family, friends, coworkers, and even perfect strangers truly can impact your success and happiness in life. If you want to be on a more even keel, try evening out your blood sugar levels.

Fewer Sick Days

Bacteria and viruses *love* sugar. They gobble it up and use it to grow and multiply. When blood sugar levels are up, the levels of sugar in virtually all of the body's tissues and fluids rise as well. That makes the diabetic body an ideal breeding ground for infection. If you ignore your high blood sugar levels, therefore, you are essentially supplying extra nutrients to the bad guys. Think of it as aiding and abetting the enemy. Everything from common colds and the flu to sinus infections and vaginal yeast

29

infections are more common when blood sugar levels are elevated. And once illnesses and infections set in, they are much more difficult to shake when blood sugar is high. In fact, people with diabetes are much more likely to die from pneumonia or influenza than are people who do not have diabetes. Research has shown that people who have better blood sugar control spend significantly fewer days absent from work, sick in bed, and restricted from their usual activities. So if you don't like getting sick, take better care of your diabetes!

Softer Skin & Healthier Gums

Two other body parts that are affected immediately by changes in blood sugar levels are the skin and gums. The softness of your skin is greatly influenced by your level of hydration. When your blood sugar is high, your body tends to become dehydrated (due to urine diuresis, discussed previously). This leads to dry, cracked skin that can be more than uncomfortable and unsightly; it can open the door to infection, since the skin is your body's first line of defense against harmful bacteria and other microbes. Maintaining your blood sugar near normal helps to prevent dehydration and keep your skin intact, soft, and supple.

Your gums are also immediately affected by changes in your blood sugar levels. Blood vessels bring oxygen-rich blood to the gum tissue to nourish it. However, if the blood has a high sugar content, that same blood flow can encourage the rapid growth of bacteria living below the gumline. After feasting on the sugar, the bacteria form plaque at an accelerated rate, contributing to bleeding gums and tooth loss. Controlling your diabetes will help reduce plaque buildup immediately.

Greater Personal Safety

Driving a car, operating machinery, crossing a street, and climbing stairs can all be dangerous, even deadly, undertakings for you and for those around you—if you have uncontrolled blood sugar levels. You've already learned how high blood sugar can cause sleepiness and slow reaction times—a recipe for disaster when driving. But the opposite extreme, **hypoglycemia,** or low blood

Hypoglycemia Defined

Hypoglycemia, commonly known as low blood sugar, means the blood sugar level is below 70 mg/dl. In hypoglycemia, certain body parts and systems are deprived of the energy they need to function properly. Hypoglycemia can occur when too much insulin is taken or when the pancreas is overstimulated by certain medications. You can usually reverse it quickly by consuming a rapid-acting carbohydrate source, such as crackers, juice, or sugary candy that has little or no fat. (The fat in chocolate slows the digestion of its sugar, making chocolate a little less effective than other sweet candy at raising blood sugar quickly.)

sugar, can be even more dangerous. It can put you in a coma and even kill you if it's not treated quickly enough.

Hypoglycemia can occur in anyone with diabetes who injects insulin or takes an oral diabetes medication that stimulates the pancreas to produce extra insulin, including a sulfonylurea (glipizide or glyburide) or a meglitinide (repaglinide or nateglinide). A blood sugar level that is below normal (defined as less than 70 mg/dl) usually causes the brain (as well as other body systems) to malfunction. Decision-making ability, judgment, and even awareness become impaired. Coordination suffers, and trembling can occur. So if you want to do all that you can to keep yourself and those around you safe, you must avoid blood sugar extremes by controlling your blood sugar levels.

STEP 3:
Remember Control's Preventive Power

There may be no better motivation for stabilizing your blood sugar than the fear of living with—or dying from—the devastating long-term complications that are likely to occur if you don't.

ANYONE WHO HAS ever owned a car knows the importance of regular oil changes. Of course, when I was in my twenties (and a bit strapped for cash), the whole idea of "preventive maintenance" seemed a bit foreign to me. Why would anyone waste their hard-earned money fixing something that wasn't broken? I even had a theory that the oil companies invented the 3,000-mile oil change just to sell more lubricant.

Then came that unforgettable winter night in northern Indiana. My wife and I were driving home to Chicago after visiting her family in Cleveland. It was a blustery night on a barren stretch of highway, and there wasn't another sign of life for miles. Out of nowhere, the red "check engine" light flickered on the dashboard. Moments later, the silence was broken by a clicking sound coming from the engine. After a few minutes, the clicks turned into loud pops, and the pops grew into deafening bangs. Before I knew what was happening, the dashboard lit up like a Christmas tree, black smoke poured from under the hood, and our little car came to a grinding halt in the middle of nowhere.

Good News!

Studies have shown that by dropping pounds and getting more active, people with pre-diabetes can delay or prevent type 2 diabetes and even return their blood sugar levels to the normal range.

This was before the age of cell phones, so we were more or less stranded until a patrol car found us and called for a tow. The next morning, we found out that the car had "blown a rod." One of the pistons had literally broken through the engine housing, splattering thick black oil everywhere. Even with my limited knowledge of the internal combustion engine, that didn't sound good. And it wasn't. The entire engine had to be replaced. It cost thousands of dollars, and by the time my wife and I got home, we each had missed a couple days of work.

All because I had not bothered to change the oil for more than a year. Sure, I saved about 20 bucks and 20 minutes of my precious time upfront, but the ultimate cost was huge. Besides losing a great deal of time and money, I put myself and my wife in what could have been a very dangerous situation.

The moral of the story: It's a lot easier to prevent problems than it is to fix them. Change the oil every few months, and you won't "blow a rod."

There are probably a thousand examples of how we follow the wisdom of prevention in our daily lives: We change the furnace filter to keep the heater working. We use a surge protector to keep from frying the television or computer. We even spray the lawn for weeds before the weeds show up. Why don't we treat our bodies to the same kind of preventive care?

Easy Diabetes Control Secret #3:
It's a lot easier to prevent problems than it is to fix them once they've developed.

We all know of someone who wound up going blind, losing a foot, or needing kidney dialysis as a result of diabetes. Unfortunately, that's only the tip of the iceberg when it comes to the long-term effects of poorly controlled diabetes. Diabetes can produce a number of serious consequences if you don't take good care of yourself and manage your condition properly.

If the thought of your body decaying and falling apart strikes serious fear into you, *good!* Fear can be a powerful motivator. It's what keeps us from doing stupid things like playing with fire and picking fights with people twice our size. And maybe, just maybe, it will inspire you to control your blood sugar.

So in this step, we'll spend some time becoming familiar with the proven long-term benefits of quality blood sugar management, including:

- Improved heart health
- Better blood flow
- Healthy kidneys
- Proper nerve function
- Less nerve pain
- Fit feet
- Clear vision
- Mental soundness
- Healthy teeth and gums
- Flexible joints
- A positive outlook

Improved Heart Health

Despite the long list of health problems diabetes can cause, heart disease is what ultimately kills the majority of people with diabetes. People with diabetes are two to four times more likely to develop heart disease and five times more likely to die from it than are people without diabetes. Why? To begin with, many people with diabetes are overweight and have elevated blood cholesterol and blood pressure levels, any one of which on its own increases the risk of heart disease. But having excess sugar in the bloodstream threatens the heart in other ways, too. Sugar is a sticky substance (think of the last time you ate cotton candy or spilled juice). It makes cholesterol, fat, and other substances in the blood stick to the interior walls of blood vessels, contributing to the formation of **plaque.** Plaque makes blood vessels thick and inflexible, a condition known as **atherosclerosis,** or hardening of the arteries. The thickening of the blood vessel walls narrows the space through which the blood flows, slowing its passage. And sometimes pieces of plaque break off, which may lead to the formation of blood clots that further restrict the flow of blood to vital organs such as the heart.

The good news: Improving blood sugar control dramatically reduces the risk of heart disease. Besides preventing the formation of much of the plaque that clogs blood vessels, better diabetes management also frequently leads to reductions in blood cholesterol and blood pressure levels. Plus, the positive lifestyle steps you take to control blood sugar, such as exercising regularly, eating more healthfully, and cutting back on stress, further reduce your risk of heart disease.

Better Blood Flow

In addition to the heart, a number of other vital body parts require large amounts of oxygen and depend on healthy blood vessels to deliver an unobstructed flow of oxygen-rich blood. The most important of these is the brain. When a blood vessel leading to the brain becomes clogged with sticky plaque, the brain cells normally fed by that vessel do not receive enough oxygen and quickly die. This is called a **stroke.** The risk of stroke is two to four times higher in people with diabetes than in those without it, and the risk more than doubles after a person has had type 2 diabetes for as little as five years.

The muscles in the legs also depend on a reliable and substantial flow of blood. When blood vessels that feed the legs become clogged, the leg muscles don't get sufficient oxygen, which can lead to pain or cramping during exercising, walking, or simply standing—a condition called **claudication.** Blood vessel disease in the legs is *twenty times* more common in people with diabetes than in those without it. Claudication occurs in 15 percent of people who have had diabetes for 10 years and 45 percent of those who have had it for 20 years.

The good news: Tightening blood sugar control, along with all the other changes and lifestyle improvements that come with it, will help blood flow more freely to all the vital body parts. For people with diabetes who have already developed circulatory problems, the news is even better: Symptoms often decrease as blood sugar levels improve.

Healthy Kidneys

Visit any kidney dialysis center and check the charts of the people who sit there for hours a day, several days a week, with tubes in their arms, hooked up to machines that filter waste products, toxins, and other undesirable substances from their blood. Diabetic. Diabetic. Not Diabetic. Diabetic. Diabetic.

Get the idea?

Diabetes is the leading cause of kidney failure, accounting for 44 percent of new cases of kidney disease. Nearly 200,000 Americans with diabetes have received kidney transplants or are receiving dialysis treatment. Approximately 50,000 Americans with diabetes begin treatment for end-stage renal (kidney) disease each year. Minorities, especially African Americans and Hispanics, who have type 2 diabetes are highly susceptible to kidney disease, but everyone with

> ### Busy Kidneys
>
> More than 2,500 pints of blood pass through your kidneys every day, an amount that would fill roughly 28 beer kegs. Every drop of blood in your body is filtered by your kidneys once an hour.

elevated blood sugar levels is at risk. Elevated blood sugar damages the tiny blood vessels, called capillaries, that form and nourish the filters within the kidneys.

The good news: Tightening blood sugar control dramatically reduces the risk of kidney disease. In fact, major studies examining the effect of blood sugar levels on kidney disease found that every 30 mg/dl drop in average blood sugar leads to a 30 percent reduction in the risk of kidney disease.

Proper Nerve Function

The nervous system is like the body's electrical wiring, relaying signals that control voluntary and involuntary functions throughout the body. A portion of that interior wiring, called the **autonomic** nervous system, controls the body's involuntary activities—all of the basic, "behind the scenes" functions, such as the beating of the heart, the digestion of food, the regulation of body temperature, the maintenance of balance, and the physical response to sexual stimulation, that occur without conscious thought or direction on our part.

Nerves are like any other living tissue in the body: They use sugar for energy, and they require an unobstructed blood supply to provide them with oxygen and other nutrients. Excess sugar in the blood appears to cause two main problems for the nervous system. First, it interferes with the blood supply to the nerves—just as it interferes with the flow of blood to other parts of the body—by contributing to plaque buildup in the blood vessel walls. Second, high blood sugar seems to alter energy metabolism (the process of using sugar to fuel cell functions) in such a way that the nerves swell and the coating on the outside of the nerve fibers fails to do its job of insulating and protecting the nerves. When the nerves that regulate basic body functions are damaged in this way by high blood sugar levels, the condition is referred to as **autonomic neuropathy.**

Population-based studies have shown that 60 to 70 percent of people with diabetes have some form of mild to severe nerve damage. For example, nearly 50 percent of all men with diabetes develop impotency within a decade of diagnosis, due mainly to malfunction of the nerves that produce an erection. Women with diabetes are more likely than women without it to suffer from vaginal dryness, again as a result of damage to nerves that control sexual response. Nerve damage can also lead to delayed digestion, a condition known as **gastroparesis** that affects upward of 30 percent of people with type 2 diabetes. Gastroparesis can cause painful bloating and, because it delays the peaking of blood sugar that normally occurs after a meal, can make diabetes even harder to control. **Postural hypotension,** yet another condition caused by damage to nerves, is twice as common in people with diabetes. It is a type of low blood pressure that occurs upon sitting or standing and can lead to dizziness and fainting.

The good news: Blood sugar control is an effective means of preventing all forms of autonomic neuropathy. And while autonomic neuropathy is not always reversible once it has developed, the condition may regress slightly or at least won't progress as quickly once blood sugar levels are returned to normal.

Less Nerve Pain

As previously mentioned, 60 to 70 percent of all people with diabetes develop some form of nerve damage in their lifetime. Of those, most develop a form called **peripheral neuropathy**—malfunction of the nerves serving the feet and lower legs. In its early stages, peripheral neuropathy expresses itself as tingling or numbness. But as it progresses and nerves become inflamed, it can cause constant and sometimes severe pain. While there are several conventional and alternative medical treatments for painful neuropathy, many sufferers find little or no relief.

The good news: Tight blood sugar control can help to minimize the pain and slow the progression of peripheral neuropathy. Even better, if it is initiated early enough in the course of diabetes, tight control may actually prevent peripheral neuropathy from developing in the first place.

Fit Feet

Yet another problem resulting from peripheral neuropathy is the risk of serious foot infections and deformities. How can a nerve problem lead to infection? It's a rather simple chain reaction. If, because of numbness, you cannot feel a minor foot injury and so continue to use that foot, the injury can grow more severe. If there is inadequate blood flow to the injured area to aid in the healing process—a likely scenario considering the circulation problems common among people with diabetes—an infection can easily develop. As the infection spreads into the underlying tissue and bone, portions of the foot suffer cell death, a condition known as **gangrene.**

Foot deformities often develop because the nerves that coordinate complex movements in the feet fail to do their job. The person with neuropathy may put pressure on inappropriate (or injured) areas of the foot and cause further damage that goes unnoticed due to the lack of pain sensation.

Each year, more than 70,000 people with diabetes require lower-limb amputations. Diabetes is the underlying reason for more amputations than all other causes combined, and loss of protective nerve sensation is the most critical factor. Even more disturbing is the fact that most people with diabetes who have a toe, foot, or limb amputated die within three years.

The good news: Tight blood sugar control helps to preserve sufficient blood flow to, and healthy nerve function in, the feet. In addition, as discussed in Step 2, lowering blood sugar levels helps to reduce the risk of infection. That's really good news for those looking to prevent foot problems as well as those recovering from existing foot ailments.

Clear Vision

In the back of the eye is a sensitive layer of tissue called the **retina** that acts like the film in a camera. The retina receives and records light from the outside world. Those images in light are then converted into electrical signals that are transmitted to the

No Guarantees

While maintaining tight control of blood sugar can greatly reduce the risk of developing serious health problems related to diabetes, there are no guarantees. So it's important to stay alert to the possible signs that a complication is developing. Early detection and treatment are key to minimizing the damage. At least once a year, see your ophthalmologist for an eye exam. Have your teeth cleaned and your gums checked for signs of periodontal disease at least twice, but preferably several times, a year. And have your feet examined and tested for adequate nerve sensation every time you visit your physician. (To remind yourself and your physician to perform this quick check, take off your shoes and socks once you're sitting in the exam room.)

brain to produce vision. A network of capillaries provides the living cells of the retina with oxygen and nutrients. Elevated blood sugar levels, however, weaken these tiny blood vessels. As a result, they may swell, leak, or grow in unhealthy ways, blocking light from ever reaching the retina. This condition is called **diabetic retinopathy.**

Diabetes is the leading cause of blindness among adults ages 20 to 74. Diabetic retinopathy accounts for approximately 20,000 new cases of blindness each year. In fact, roughly one of every five people with type 2 diabetes already has retinopathy when they are diagnosed with diabetes. Glaucoma, cataracts, and diseases of the cornea (the transparent outer covering of the eyeball) are also more common in people with diabetes and contribute to the high rate of blindness among this population.

The good news: Tight blood sugar control reduces the risk of retinopathy. Every 30 mg/dl reduction in average blood sugar lowers the risk of retinopathy by approximately 30 percent. For those with existing retinopathy, tightening blood sugar control slows the progression significantly.

Mental Soundness

With aging comes increased risk for a number of health problems. Few instill as much fear as Alzheimer's disease, a progressive and ultimately fatal disease that destroys brain cells, causing increasingly severe problems with memory, thinking, and behavior along the way. Today, it affects more than five million Americans and is the sixth-leading cause of death in the United States. Currently, there is no cure for Alzheimer's. Damaged blood vessels in the brain are believed to play a role in the development of Alzheimer's, and uncontrolled type 2 diabetes greatly increases the risk of the disease.

The good news: If you have type 2 diabetes, tight blood sugar control can reduce your risk of Alzheimer's disease to that of the general nondiabetic population.

Healthy Teeth & Gums

Adults with diabetes have two times the risk of developing gum disease (periodontitis) as do their peers without diabetes. Almost one-third of people with diabetes have severe gum disease. Specifically, those with type 2 diabetes have greater plaque buildup and more bacteria below the gumline; as a result, their gums bleed more easily, and they commonly experience loosening and loss of teeth. Once a gum infection starts, it can take a long time to eradicate it when blood sugar is out of whack. Conversely, research has shown that having periodontal disease may make it more difficult for people who have diabetes to control their blood sugar levels.

The good news: Good blood sugar control can help prevent dental problems. The lower the average blood sugar level, the lower the risk of gum disease and tooth loss.

Flexible Joints

Joint mobility problems, including conditions such as frozen shoulder, trigger finger, and clawing of the hand, affect approximately 20 percent of people with diabetes, and high blood sugar is the root cause. Excess sugar in the blood sticks to collagen, a protein found in bone, cartilage, and tendons. When collagen becomes sugar-coated, it thickens and stiffens, preventing joints from moving smoothly through their full range of motion and often causing joint pain.

The good news: Keeping your blood sugar levels near normal reduces your risk of developing joint mobility problems. And if you already have limited range of motion in your shoulders, hands, fingers, or other joints, lowering your blood sugar levels may help improve your range of motion and limit the pain associated with stiff joints.

A Positive Outlook

Blood sugar levels have a direct effect on our mental well-being. It is common for people with diabetes to feel down when their blood sugar levels are up. Depression is three times more common in adults with diabetes than in the general population. The mechanism of this increased risk is not entirely known. Since depression is often biochemical in nature, elevated sugar levels in the brain may play a direct role. It could also be related to the extra stress associated with living with a chronic illness. Certainly, developing complications from diabetes can instill a feeling of helplessness, a definite contributing factor in the onset of depression.

The good news: Improving your blood sugar levels can make you a happier person. Researchers at Harvard Medical School and the Joslin Diabetes Center studied the effects of blood sugar control on mood and disposition. They found that people with lower blood sugar levels reported a higher overall quality of life. Significantly better ratings were given in the areas of physical, emotional, and general health and vitality.

So that's pretty much the situation. Almost every aspect of your physical and mental well-being is influenced by your blood sugar levels. Improving your blood sugar control will enable you to feel and perform better today and enjoy a healthier and more comfortable life for many tomorrows.

STEP 4:
Develop an Attitude

To succeed in recapturing control of your blood sugar levels, you must adopt a state of mind that says, "I will do whatever it takes, no matter what."

THINK ABOUT THE jobs you've held in your lifetime and the bosses and supervisors you've worked for over the years. Chances are you have fond memories of some and less positive memories of others. Supervising a small staff of my own, I've tried to learn what it takes to be a good supervisor. One thing that comes up in virtually every management book I've read and seminar I've attended is this: A good supervisor makes work seem as little like work as possible.

That doesn't mean employees are allowed to play all day. Rather, it means a good supervisor realizes that everyone needs to feel they are part of an important and worthwhile effort, a cause greater than their specific job. From the most mundane task to the most challenging, everything gets done faster and better when everyone believes in that larger purpose.

Here's a good example. Some years ago, heavy rains in the Midwest led to historic flooding in towns all along the Mississippi River Valley. Thousands of people from across the country, many with no link whatsoever to the people affected by the floods, met in the country's midsection to dig trenches, fill and stack sandbags, and do whatever was necessary to divert the onslaught of muddy water. It was exhausting work, both mentally and physically. And the payment for providing hours, days, and, in some cases, weeks of tireless labor consisted of little more than coffee, soggy sandwiches, and the gratitude of residents.

So what was it that enticed all those people to go there and do what they did? What kept them going when they were cold, wet, dirty, and tired? Attitude. The attitude that it was the right thing to do and nothing was going to get in the way of doing it. Win or lose, they were determined to do all they could to help. And that's just what they did.

Easy Diabetes Control Secret #4:
Every job is easier when you've got the right attitude.

When it comes to taking control of your diabetes, it is just as important to develop the right attitude from the get-go. Is it fair that your body does not process sugar properly? Is it fair that you have to go through all these trials and tribulations to manage your blood sugar? Is it fair that you're at risk of losing your eyes, kidneys, and feet because of your disease? Heck no! And yes, you deserve to be angry. But rather than allowing the anger to become a weight around your neck, funnel that emotion and energy into developing a serious attitude. Make it 100 percent

Make a List, Check It Often

It takes more than good intentions to control your blood sugar. Without a solid plan and appropriate follow-through, the chances of success are pretty slim. This book provides an easy, step-by-step path to blood sugar control. And the list of those steps printed below can help remind you to follow through. Photocopy it, tape the copy to your fridge, and check it often. You'll be amazed at the feeling of accomplishment you'll get as you progress through the list. Just be sure you don't skip any steps. Do them in the order listed; they're far easier to accomplish that way.

The Easy Path to Control

1. Know your opponent.

2. Focus on control's immediate benefits.

3. Remember control's preventive power.

4. Develop an attitude.

5. Set your targets.

6. Test your blood sugar levels.

7. Prepare to unleash your lifestyle tools.

8. Get moving.

9. Manage stress.

10. Eat for control.

11. Call in the cavalry.

clear in your mind that controlling your blood sugar is the right thing to do—diabetes will *not* get the best of you!—and *nothing* is going to get in your way.

As we have already discussed, diabetes is deadly serious stuff. Whether you have had diabetes for years, were recently diagnosed, have been classified as "pre-diabetic," or are simply at high risk for the disease, the whole issue of having a major metabolic system breaking down deserves serious attention. Based on my years of experience working in the diabetes field, I can honestly say that the number one reason diabetes causes so many health problems is that most people who have it just don't take it seriously enough. But once you develop the right attitude, that won't be a problem for you.

One trick I've learned is to write down things I want to commit to. For some reason, putting a commitment in writing is like stamping it in permanent ink onto your soul. Here's an example:

> I am going to control my diabetes, and nothing is going to stand in my way.

Now you try. You don't have to use the same phrasing. Use your own words to inscribe, in the box below, your commitment to yourself and your health and well-being.

And what about the whole issue of not letting things "stand in the way"? What *could* get in the way?

There are many hurdles you will face in your efforts to control your blood sugar. You cannot avoid them. But you can be prepared to deal with the obstacles, and you can jump over them (or plow right through them, if you prefer).

For example, costs are often an obstacle. Many people let out-of-pocket expenses get in the way of taking proper care of themselves. As one of my previous clients put it, "If my health insurance doesn't pay for it, I don't need it." Hogwash! Does health insurance pay for the food you put on your table? The clothes you wear? The air you breathe? Health insurance is really designed to offset major medical expenses, the kind that would bankrupt most people. You need to be prepared to absorb at least some of the cost associated with the tools of day-to-day diabetes management, such as medications, health education, exercise equipment, and so on. Look at these expenses as investments in yourself and your future. You can pay a few bucks now to meet with a registered dietitian and develop a good meal plan, or you can fork over a whole lot more down the road for coronary bypass surgery, when the years of neglecting your health finally catch up with you. Remember: You can't take it with you!

Of course, there is nothing wrong with looking for some help to pay for necessary medications and supplies. (I happen to be the ultimate bargain hunter!) One place you might start is the Foundation for Health Coverage Education, a nonprofit that helps people without health insurance to locate public and private assistance programs. You can visit their Web site at www.coverageforall.org or call them toll-free at 1-800-234-1317 to discuss your options with a specialist.

Another possible obstacle may include family and friends. They can sometimes put you in situations that make it difficult (if not impossible) for you to stick to your diabetes management program. Schedules may get out-of-kilter, food choices may not be optimal, and time for physical activity may become curtailed. And we all know how much stress those closest to us can cause!

The important thing to remember is that this is *your* diabetes, *your* health, *your* life—not theirs. Let them do what they want; it's not your job (nor is it possible, for that matter) to change the way others live their lives. All you can do is make the right choices for yourself. And if you are concerned about how others will view you for adopting a healthier lifestyle, stop worrying. Deep down, everyone respects and admires those who make the tough choices and take good care of themselves, as long as they don't try to force their beliefs on others.

So the next time your family comes together for a holiday, don't hesitate to get up from the sofa and politely ask, "Anyone care to join me for a walk?" If nobody joins you, that's okay. Maybe next time someone will be inspired by what you're doing and tag along. And the next time you get together with your friends for a game of bridge or rummy, remember that there is no rule stating that you must consume a handful of snacks for every hand of cards. Have fun, and enjoy the camaraderie and challenge of the game. Just do so without stuffing yourself.

Family and friends can also be a source of many, many questions that you may not care to answer. "Should you be eating that?" "Why do you have to check your blood sugar so much?" "Did you get diabetes from eating too much sugar?" Having dealt with such questions myself since I was diagnosed with diabetes more than 20 years ago, take my advice: Answer their questions. The more your friends and family know about your disease, the more likely they will be to accept and support your management efforts. The less they know, the more likely they will misunderstand and come to false conclusions. So show off your knowledge! Take the opportunity to teach others what you have learned.

Life can also create obstacles to taking good care of your health. Work demands, family obligations, social commitments, household responsibilities, and unforeseen developments can threaten your best-laid diabetes control plans. That's when prioritizing becomes essential. As part of the attitude you've adopted, you

It's a Family Affair

Diabetes is sometimes referred to as a family disease, because it tends to affect every family member to some extent. It may alter food selection and preparation and timing of family meals. It may affect family leisure time (less TV, more physical activity). It may affect family finances. And it's likely to spark an array of emotions—from worry to resentment. To help your family cope with the adjustments, teach them as much as you can about diabetes, encourage them to voice their questions and emotions, and involve them in your quest for good control. Share your treatment plan with them, explain why meal planning and blood testing are so vital, tutor them on how to recognize and react to signs of hypoglycemia, and provide concrete suggestions for how they can support you. After all, diabetes is a family affair.

need to make diabetes self-care a high priority in your life. That's not to say that you should neglect other important aspects of your life, but you need to find ways to incorporate diabetes self-care no matter how full your days become.

For example, several of my busy clients find it challenging to fit exercise into their day, but they manage. Some reserve a specific time in their daily schedule for exercise, actually blocking off the time in their personal or business planner the way they would for an important meeting. Others find ways to multitask by sneaking in exercise as they handle other demands. A few have even cut back on their work responsibilities to make time for their own health benefit.

One other obstacle that could get in the way of doing what you need to do is your self-image—your view of who you are and what you stand for. You may never have thought of yourself as an "active person," a "healthy eater," or even a "person who is beating diabetes." *That needs to change.* The moment you start thinking of yourself in terms like these, that's when good things are going to start happening for you.

STEP 5:
Set Your Targets

To know where you stand right now and where you want to go in terms of blood sugar control, you need tools for measuring your progress and goals that will tell you when you've arrived.

SUCCESS MEANS DIFFERENT things to different people. Take my friend John, for example. John works for the local police department. He's trying to move up the ladder to the position of lieutenant. He has to pass written tests in order to receive a promotion, but there is much more to it than that.

In John's mind, he should be viewed by his superiors as a quality officer based on his job performance: how many "bad guys" he puts away, how well he works with other officers and the public, his safety record, and so on. He focuses on being the best street cop he can be. He works long hours (including many of the shifts his colleagues don't like to work), studies hard, and conducts himself professionally. He doesn't always dot his i's and cross his t's, but he gets results.

During his recent review, however, John found out that he was being passed over for promotion. Why? Because he has been routinely late turning in his weekly reports. Apparently, paperwork is very important to his superiors. And if your paperwork doesn't get done on time and in proper order, you're not going anywhere in that department. Your name could be Columbo and it wouldn't matter. To the powers that be, Dirty Harry just doesn't make a good manager.

So John learned a valuable lesson: If you want to do a good job, you'd better find out how "good" is defined.

Easy Diabetes Control Secret #5:
It's easier to succeed if you know the definition of success.

To successfully manage diabetes, quality blood sugar control is the gold standard. To even have a shot at meeting that standard, however, you first need to be able to track your blood sugar and gauge your level of control. That requires two tools: individual blood sugar readings and HbA1c measurements.

Individual Blood Sugar Readings

Individual blood sugar readings are essential for evaluating your blood sugar control (or lack thereof). These are the readings you get by pricking your finger to obtain a small drop of blood, which you place on a testing strip that you insert into a portable blood glucose meter. The meter then measures and reports your blood sugar reading at that specific time. Such immediate information not only provides you with a tool for tracking your control, it allows you to take immediate action to bring a high or low level back into a healthier range.

Of course, blood sugar levels naturally vary throughout the day and from day to day, depending on a variety of factors, such as when you ate your last meal, took your diabetes medication, or exercised. By taking multiple readings each day and then averaging together all of the readings from the last one or two weeks, you can get additional insight into your level of control. (Indeed, some glucose meters automatically calculate the average of your recent readings for you.)

However, *quality* blood sugar control doesn't just mean having the lowest average. It also requires stability, because blood sugar readings that bounce from high to low aren't healthy, even when they result in an average that doesn't look so bad. Consider, for example, the following two people:

	Blood Sugars	**Average**
Fred	113, 97, 120, 135, 144, 100, 177, 83, 111	120
Barney	53, 204, 188, 67, 170, 68, 80, 202, 48	120

Both men have the same average blood sugar level. But look at the *variation* in Barney's readings: His blood sugar is high half the time and low half the time. Fred's blood sugar levels, on the other hand, are more stable and consistent, with no wild upward or downward spikes.

Too much variability in blood sugar levels can affect a person's quality of life. Having an episode of low blood sugar can be dangerous as well as uncomfortable, because it can cause symptoms such as dizziness, weakness, and rapid heartbeat; left untreated, it can quickly lead to blurred vision, confusion, loss of consciousness, and coma. Experiencing such risky lows on a regular basis is like living life on a tightrope. A high level of blood sugar, conversely, saps energy and mental focus, and frequent highs can become a real drag on the body and mind. There is also evidence that excessive variability in blood sugar levels can cause damage to blood vessels, even if the overall average is within the preferred range.

The preferred, or ideal, range for your blood sugar level depends on your current diabetes treatment regimen and how likely it is to cause hypoglycemia, or low blood sugar (see Risky Business on page 62). That ideal range also varies based on when you take a reading—your ideal range will be different after a night of fasting than it will be an hour or two after a meal, for example. You can use the table on page 63 to determine your ideal fasting,

Risky Business

Many older diabetes medications force the pancreas to secrete extra insulin regardless of the blood sugar level and can therefore cause hypoglycemia, or low blood sugar. These medications include the ones listed below as well as any combination pills that contain any of these medications:

- tolbutamide (Orinase)
- acetohexamide (Dymelor)
- tolazamide (Tolinase)
- chlorpropamide (Diabinese)
- glipizide (Glucotrol)
- glyburide (Diabeta, Micronase, Glynase)
- glimepiride (Amaryl)
- gliclazide (Diamicron)
- repaglinide (Prandin)
- nateglinide (Starlix)

pre-meal, and post-meal ranges. Once you know them, you can assess the quality of your blood sugar control by considering how often your readings fall within the appropriate ranges.

It is not necessary for your blood sugar to be in your ideal range every time you check it. We all have moments of weakness when it comes to taking care of our diabetes. As a general rule, if at

IDEAL BLOOD SUGAR RANGES

	Fasting (Wake-Up) Range	Pre-Meal Range	Post-Meal Range (1–2 Hours After Eating)
No risk of hypoglycemia*	70–100 mg/dl	70–120 mg/dl	<140 mg/dl
Low risk of hypoglycemia**	70–120 mg/dl	70–140 mg/dl	<160 mg/dl
High risk of hypoglycemia***	80–140 mg/dl	80–160 mg/dl	<180 mg/dl

* Includes those who are not taking insulin or medications that can cause hypoglycemia (glyburide, glipizide, meglitinides).

** Includes those taking insulin once daily or oral medications that can cause hypoglycemia (glyburide, glipizide, meglitinides).

*** Includes those taking multiple insulin injections daily and those unable to detect hypoglycemia.

least 75 percent (three-fourths) of your readings are in the proper range, you're doing a pretty good job of controlling your blood sugar. If more than 10 percent of your readings are below your ideal range or if more than 25 percent are above it, you may need some additional self-management education or an adjustment to your medication regime.

Consider Betty, for example. She does not take any medication that can cause hypoglycemia, so her ideal pre-meal range is 70 to 120. The following are her blood sugar readings for five days:

M	TU	W	TH	F
104	174	138	97	86
225	126	125	101	99
166	213	159	110	90
113	98	79	185	143

Out of 20 readings, none is below her ideal range, which is good; however, 10 are above the upper limit of 120. That means 50 percent of her readings are above her ideal range. So Betty needs to work on tightening her pre-meal blood sugar control.

If your current blood sugar readings are well above your ideal ranges, it's reasonable to set temporary targets that fall between the two. For example, if you are not at risk for hypoglycemia but have blood sugars that are consistently above 200, an initial goal might be to get your readings into the 100 to 180 range. Once you've brought your sugar levels down into that target range, you can then aim for your ideal range(s).

HbA1c Measurements

The second essential tool for gauging your blood sugar control is a test that measures glycohemoglobin A1c, often referred to as HbA1c or simply A1c. The result of this simple blood test, arranged through your doctor's office, reflects your average blood sugar level over the previous two to three months, giving you insight into your blood sugar control over a longer term.

Why Bother Checking A1c?

Since the A1c result reflects your average blood sugar level over the previous two to three months, why not just average the results of your individual blood sugar (finger-stick) tests for that period instead? Because it doesn't work. Averaging your finger-stick readings over a three-month period almost always underestimates the true average blood sugar level as determined through the A1c test. There are several reasons why this occurs. Most people test their blood sugar before they eat, when blood sugars are at their low point, rather than after they eat, when blood sugars naturally run higher. There is also a tendency to perform the finger-stick test more frequently when blood sugars are running low, and these additional low readings tend to artificially skew the average lower. Finally, in many people, blood sugars rise in the middle of the night, a time when blood sugars are rarely checked; these highs don't get factored into an average that is calculated using only the results of individual daytime blood tests.

Inside your red blood cells is a protein called hemoglobin that carries oxygen from your lungs to your body's tissues. Sugar in the blood has a tendency to glycate, or stick to, this protein, forming glycohemoglobin. Once the glucose attaches to the hemoglobin, it stays there as long as the red blood cell lives, typically two to three months. Your red blood cells don't all die at once; old ones are constantly dying, and new ones are constantly being created. So at any one time, your red blood cells are a mix of the very old, the middle aged, and the quite young.

In someone without diabetes, roughly 4 to 6 percent of their hemoglobin is coated with sugar. In the person with diabetes, whose blood sugar levels are higher, more sugar attaches to the hemoglobin molecules; usually anywhere from 6 to more than 20 percent of the hemoglobin is sugar-coated. The A1c test measures this percentage. (A1c, by the way, refers to a type of glucose-coated hemoglobin that is especially suited for gauging long-term blood sugar levels.) And because some of the hemoglobin molecules in the blood are older and some newer, the A1c result provides a good estimate of how high the blood sugar has been over the past two to three months.

Using the results from the A1c and at-home blood sugar tests provides a fuller and more accurate picture of your level of control. Using the at-home results alone would be like trying to judge a baseball batter's ability by looking at a day or two of single at-bats. Just as a great hitter will make an out or have a bad day sometimes, a person with good control will have the occasional high or low. So to truly gauge the player's batting skill, you need to also see his season average. And to really evaluate your level of sugar control, you need to know your A1c.

To translate your A1c result into an average blood sugar level, you can use the following formula:

$$(A1c \times 28.7) - 46.7 = \text{average blood sugar}$$

Or, if math isn't your thing, just use this table:

A1c	Average blood sugar
5%	97
6%	126
7%	154
8%	183
9%	212
10%	240
11%	269
12%	298
13%	326
14%	355

There's another reason testing A1c is so important. Research has shown it is closely linked to the risk of developing diabetic complications. Essentially, the higher the A1c, the greater the risk of developing eye, kidney, nerve, and heart problems. That is why efforts should be made to keep the A1c as near to normal as possible. In most cases, that equates to an A1c of 6 to 7 percent. A looser A1c of 7 to 8 percent, however, may be a more appropriate target for anyone in whom an episode of hypoglycemia would be especially dangerous, including:

- Anyone who is susceptible to low blood sugar but suffers from hypoglycemia unawareness, a condition in which the individual is unable to detect the warning symptoms of a dropping blood sugar level until it is too late for them to help themselves; it can develop in people who have had diabetes for many years.

- Anyone who has significant heart disease (the rapid heartbeat and overall physical stress placed on the body during an episode of hypoglycemia can be particularly dangerous for a person who has an already weakened heart).

- Anyone who works in an extremely high-risk profession, where experiencing dizziness, blurred vision, confusion, or loss of consciousness due to hypoglycemia could be devastating (picture a construction worker walking across a roofing beam or a window washer laboring on the side of a skyscraper, for example).

- A very young child who cannot communicate symptoms of hypoglycemia.

On the other hand, a tighter A1c target of 5 to 6 percent may be appropriate for women who are pregnant or preparing to become pregnant, individuals planning for surgery, and anyone looking to slow or reverse existing diabetes complications.

> ## Join the Minority
>
> In 2004, only about one out of four people with diabetes had what the American Diabetes Association considers "good" control—an A1c below 7 percent. That means that about three out of four people with diabetes had an A1c level at or above 7 percent. There's just no excuse for so many people having suboptimal control! Fortunately, with the help of this step-by-step guide, you *can*, and *will*, do better.

Keep in mind that achieving these A1c targets may take time, especially if your current A1c is very high. Since the test is usually done every three months, it is reasonable to aim for an A1c that's one or two percentage points lower at each test.

Your Specific Target Ranges

When you put it all together, your ideal aim is to have the lowest possible individual blood sugar and A1c levels without experi-

encing frequent or severe hypoglycemia. Occasional, mild episodes of low blood sugar are acceptable and not dangerous for
most people with diabetes. However, if low blood sugars become
too frequent (occurring more than two or three times a week) or
severe (causing seizures or loss of consciousness), you'll need to
ease up on your targets.

Now it's time to set your own specific targets, using the information and tables in this step. Be sure to discuss them with your
doctor and other members of your diabetes care team. Then
write them in the box below so that you can easily refer to them
as you work through the remaining steps and move closer to your
goal of better control.

My Ideal Blood Sugar Ranges:

Fasting Range	Pre-Meal Range	Post-Meal Range
(upon waking)	(right before eating)	(1–2 hrs. after eating)

My A1c Target: _____%

STEP 6:
Test Your Blood Sugar Levels

You've set your sights on controlling your blood sugar. You've even specified exactly where you want your blood sugar levels to be. Now it's time to see where you actually stand.

MONITORING YOUR BLOOD sugar when you have, or are at high risk for, diabetes is very much like paying attention when you drive. You look ahead so you can assess the conditions of the road and avoid other cars. You steal quick glances at the speedometer so you can maintain a safe speed and avoid costly tickets (and accidents). And you heed the various warning lights on the dashboard so you'll know when it's time to take your vehicle in for repairs or maintenance.

Ignoring your blood sugar levels, on the other hand, is like driving with a blindfold on. Sooner or later, you're going to crash, and you might take some innocent bystanders down with you.

Properly managing diabetes means you will have to make many important choices every day. Having a sense of where you stand will help guide your decision-making.

Knowing your blood sugar "numbers" serves several important purposes:

1. It provides a measuring stick for assessing your current state of blood sugar control.

2. It lets you track your progress from one point in time to another.

3. It reveals where improvements need to be made.

4. It teaches you the impact of your daily activities and choices. You can see, almost immediately, what works and what doesn't when it comes to keeping your blood sugar in a healthy range.

Easy Diabetes Control Secret #6:
Having the right information makes it easier to make the right decisions.

As discussed in Step 5, two types of tests are used for gauging blood sugar control: The HbA1c (for measuring long-term control) and daily blood sugar readings (for measuring the sugar level and assessing control at specific moments in time). The A1c part is relatively simple to accomplish. You ask your doctor to order this test for you every three months until your sugar levels and A1c are stable and within your target ranges. Once you've reached those goals, it's usually sufficient to have the A1c test every six months (unless your physician advises more frequent tests).

Several companies offer at-home A1c test kits, but you're probably better off having a professional draw your blood and send it to a laboratory for testing. (Many doctors' offices and virtually all hospitals can do this for you.) Although the at-home kits are reasonably accurate, they require multiple steps and a much larger blood sample than that required for a typical blood sugar test. And if any of the steps are not performed exactly right, the test will be useless and you'll have wasted your money on the cost of the kit.

My First Meter

Blood sugar meters have come a long way. The first meter I used, some 25 years ago, was about the size of a brick. It required 10 microliters of blood and took more than two minutes for a single test, it had no memory, and it used test strips that had to be "blotted" halfway through the test. Today, my meter is about the size of a cell phone; has a big, bright screen; performs a blood sugar test in five seconds; and needs less than half a microliter of blood for a single test (that's twenty times less blood than my first meter required!). It stores 400 readings, provides averages, and can be hooked to a computer so that my testing data can be downloaded and further analyzed using a software program. If it could just remind me of my wife's birthday and our anniversary, it would be perfect!

Help at Your Fingertips

If you ever have trouble with your blood sugar meter, call the toll-free number located on the back of the machine. Every meter manufacturer offers a 24-hour toll-free hotline for its meter customers. Call the hotline if you have questions about proper testing procedure, are concerned about the accuracy of any readings, experience difficulties with the meter, discover that a part is missing or broken, or want to learn how to use any of your meter's advanced features (including memory recall or downloading).

So let the professionals handle this test.

As far as blood sugar testing, there are a number of elements to consider: which type of equipment to use, when to test, what to record, and, ultimately, what to do with the data.

Choosing & Using Testing Supplies

To perform the blood sugar monitoring that is so essential to good control, you need three main supplies: a blood glucose meter, the testing strips for that meter, and a lancet or lancing device to draw the small amount of blood you'll need for testing. You will also need instruction in using the supplies you choose. Your doctor, certified diabetes educator, and/or pharmacist can give you a hands-on demonstration to ensure that you are using your equipment properly. Meter manufacturers also typically have hotlines that consumers can access in order to get answers and advice about their specific meters. Take advantage of these resources so that you can confidently and correctly measure your blood sugar levels as often as necessary for good control.

When it comes to choosing a meter, remember that quality diabetes management requires accurate and frequent blood sugar testing. Selecting a meter with the desirable qualities listed below should help make *frequent* testing less of a hassle.

- Fast (some take as little as five seconds to produce a reading)

- Simple to use (fewer steps mean a quicker process and less chance for user error)

- Provides downloadable results (making it quick and easy to share your results with your diabetes care team)

- Requires very little blood (1 microliter or less is ideal)

- Easy to read (Especially if you are visually impaired, choose a meter with a very large display or one that "talks.")

The accuracy of just about every blood sugar meter on the market is pretty good. The values these meters produce typically fall within 15 percent of the reading a laboratory would produce on a blood sample taken at the same time. That's true, however, only if you use the correct testing technique. In the table on pages 76–77 are some of the more common monitoring miscues, along with explanations and solutions.

Issue	Specifics	Solution
Insufficient blood	If not enough blood is applied to the test area on the strip, the reading may be artificially low.	Dose the strip adequately, as the meter manufacturer instructs. If you suspect a strip contained too little blood, ignore the result and start over with a new strip.
Improper coding	For most meters, you must enter a code number or chip/strip for each new vial or box of strips. If the meter is not coded for that specific package of strips, the readings may be inaccurate.	Every time you begin a new box or vial of strips, code your meter according to the manufacturer's instructions.
Outdated strips	Using test strips that are outdated may produce inaccurate readings.	Check the expiration date before buying and again before starting a vial or box of strips.

Issue	Specifics	Solution
Heat or humidity	Heat and humidity will cause test strips to spoil and produce false readings.	Keep your strips sealed in their packaging and away from extreme temperatures. Do not leave test strips in your vehicle!
Dirt/impurities	Having substances like food or grease on your finger or other test site will impact the readings.	Ensure that your test site is clean when you check your blood sugar.

With the advent of alternate-site testing—using meters that can test blood taken from places other than the sensitive fingertips, such as the forearm—virtually pain-free blood sugar testing has become a reality. But be aware that alternate-site testing can be difficult with meters that require 1 microliter of blood or more. Also, a reading taken from the arm or leg may lag several minutes behind a reading taken from the fingertip. So if you suspect that your blood sugar is dropping quickly (after exercise or if you feel hypoglycemic) or rising quickly (after meals), blood taken from your fingertip will provide a more accurate reading than will a sample taken from an alternate site.

To make it more likely that you will perform the frequent blood sugar testing that is so conducive to good control, you may find it helpful to have more than one meter. Having multiple identical meters makes testing more convenient (you can keep one in the kitchen and one in the bedroom, for example, or one at work and one at home) and ensures that if one of your meters isn't functioning or gets misplaced, you will have an equivalent backup available. Some meter companies will even send you an extra meter at no charge in an effort to win your loyalty and keep you purchasing their test strips (they make their money off the strips). Personally, I keep a meter in all the places I do the most testing: bedside, kitchen, desk at work, and gym bag. I don't keep one in the car, because test strips can spoil easily at very high and low temperatures. Instead, I have an additional meter I use for traveling; I carry it with me or slip it in my briefcase to test my blood sugar before I begin driving.

When choosing a device for drawing your blood, you'll also want to opt for features and methods that will encourage—or at least won't discourage—frequent testing. For example:

- Use the thinnest-gauge lancet you can find. Presently, 33-gauge lancets are the thinnest on the market (the higher the gauge, the thinner the lancet). Thin lancets are less painful and cause less scarring than thicker lancets. Change the lancet at least once a day so the tip doesn't become dull.

- Use a lancing pen that allows you to adjust the depth of the stick, and turn it to the lightest possible setting that still produces a sufficient blood sample for your meter.

- For finger-stick testing, prick the side of your fingertip rather than the fleshy pad on the front. To obtain a sufficient blood drop after pricking, "milk" your finger by squeezing it, starting at the base and moving toward the tip.

- Opt for alternate-site testing (using your arm or leg, for example) whenever appropriate. It is almost always less painful than the finger-stick, and the readings taken at alternate sites are accurate as long as your blood sugar is not rising or dropping quickly at the time of the blood draw.

Before you go out and buy a meter at a local pharmacy, ask your doctor or diabetes educator if they have any free samples. Most meter manufacturers provide free sample meters for distribution to patients, in the hope that more patients will choose their meters and purchase their test strips for years to come. (It's like giving you a razor so that you will buy the razor blades). Most health insurance programs, including Medicare, Medicaid, and private insurance, cover the costs of meters, test strips, and lancets. You might want to consider using a reputable mail-order pharmacy or diabetes supply service; such operations will typically coordinate the insurance paperwork and ship your supplies to you as needed.

Deciding How Often to Test

When it comes to blood sugar monitoring, nobody wants to do more work than is necessary. But at the same time, it's essential that you gather enough data so you can assess the quality of your blood sugar control and do some fine-tuning of your management efforts. It is simply not sufficient to check your blood sugar only once a week or only when you wake up in the morning; you'll miss too much important information.

What follows are my testing recommendations, which vary based on whether or not you have already been diagnosed with type 2 diabetes and which, if any, diabetes medications you currently take. Find the schedule that applies to your current situation, and review the schedule with your diabetes care team before proceeding. (Be sure to read the section on record keeping later in this step, as well.)

For those with pre-diabetes or those at high risk who take no diabetes medications

This testing schedule is for those diagnosed with pre-diabetes or with a high risk of developing diabetes who do not use any oral or injectable medications or insulin for their condition.

Each week, you should test your blood sugar four times: just before breakfast one day, just before lunch another day, just before dinner on a third day, and at bedtime on a fourth day. The following is an example of how you might set up this schedule:

Sunday: No testing required.

Monday: Test before breakfast.

Tuesday: No testing required.

Wednesday: Test before lunch.

Thursday: No testing required.

Friday: Test before dinner.

Saturday: Test at bedtime.

This schedule of testing will help you and your diabetes care team to determine if your blood sugar remains in a healthy range throughout the day.

For those with type 2 diabetes who don't take insulin

This testing schedule is for those who have been diagnosed with type 2 diabetes but who do not take any insulin for their condition. This schedule applies whether or not any oral medication or injectable incretin (exenatide or pramlintide) is also being used.

Test your blood sugar every other day as follows: just before breakfast and then one to two hours after breakfast on day one, just before lunch and then one to two hours after lunch on day three, just before dinner and then one to two hours after dinner on day five, just before breakfast and one to two hours after breakfast on day seven, and so on. The following is an example of how you might set up this schedule:

Monday: Test before and one to two hours after breakfast.

Tuesday: No testing required.

Wednesday: Test before and one to two hours after lunch.

Thursday: No testing required.

Friday: Test before and one to two hours after dinner.

Saturday: No testing required.

Sunday: Test before and one to two hours after breakfast.

Monday: No testing required.

This testing schedule will allow you and your diabetes care team to see if your blood sugar remains normal before and after each of your meals. The wake-up and other pre-meal readings indicate whether your body is able to make enough of its own **basal insulin,** the baseline amount of insulin needed to offset the sugar that's naturally released by the liver between meals to maintain basic bodily functions. The after-meal readings indicate whether your pancreas can make enough **bolus insulin,** the additional burst of insulin needed at mealtimes to offset the carbohydrates from a meal.

For those with type 2 diabetes who take long-acting but not rapid-acting insulin

This testing schedule is for those who have been diagnosed with type 2 diabetes who are currently taking long-acting insulin (glargine, detemir, or NPH) but no rapid-acting (lispro, aspart, or glulisine) or pre-mixed (50/50, 70/30, or 75/25) insulin. This schedule applies whether or not any oral medication or injectable incretin (exenatide or pramlintide) is also being used.

Test your blood sugar at least twice a day, six days a week, as follows: On the first day, test just before and one to two hours after breakfast; on the second day, test just before and one to two hours after lunch; on the third day, test just before and one to two hours after dinner and also at bedtime if it follows dinner by more than three hours; and on days four through six, repeat the schedule from days one through three. Take a break from testing on the last day of each week. The following is an example of how you might set up this schedule:

Monday: Test before and one to two hours after breakfast.

Tuesday: Test before and one to two hours after lunch.

Wednesday: Test before and one to two hours after dinner and at bedtime (if it's more than three hours after dinner).

Thursday: Test before and one to two hours after breakfast.

Friday: Test before and one to two hours after lunch.

Saturday: Test before and one to two hours after dinner and at bedtime (if it's more than three hours after dinner).

Sunday: No testing required.

This testing schedule will allow you and your diabetes care team to see if your blood sugar remains normal before and after each of your meals.

For those with type 2 diabetes who take pre-mixed insulin twice a day

This testing schedule is for those who have been diagnosed with type 2 diabetes who currently inject pre-mixed insulin (50/50, 70/30, or 75/25) twice each day rather than injecting long-acting (glargine, detemir, or NPH) and/or rapid-acting (lispro, aspart, or glulisine) insulin separately. This schedule applies whether or not any oral medication or injectable incretin (exenatide or pramlintide) is also being used.

Each day of the week, test your blood sugar upon waking (before breakfast), at midday (before lunch), late in the afternoon (before dinner), and at bedtime. Also, as part of your weekly testing regimen, test your blood sugar one to two hours after breakfast on one day, one to two hours after lunch on another day, and one to two hours after dinner on a third day. The following is an example of how you might set up this schedule:

Sunday: Test before breakfast, before lunch, before dinner, and at bedtime.

Monday: Test before breakfast, one to two hours after breakfast, before lunch, before dinner, and at bedtime.

Tuesday: Test before breakfast, before lunch, before dinner, and at bedtime.

Wednesday: Test before breakfast, before lunch, one to two hours after lunch, before dinner, and at bedtime.

Thursday: Test before breakfast, before lunch, before dinner, and at bedtime.

Friday: Test before breakfast, before lunch, before dinner, one to two hours after dinner, and at bedtime.

Saturday: Test before breakfast, before lunch, before dinner, and at bedtime.

The pre-meal checks are necessary because they allow you and your diabetes care team to evaluate the effectiveness of your insulin doses. The post-meal checks help you and your team to determine the optimal timing of your two daily injections.

For those with type 2 diabetes who take insulin at each meal

This testing schedule is for those who have been diagnosed with type 2 diabetes who currently inject rapid-acting insulin (lispro, aspart, or glulisine) at each meal and use long-acting insulin (glargine, detemir, or NPH) to cover their basal insulin needs. (No pre-mixed insulin is used.) This schedule applies whether or not any oral medication or injectable incretin (exenatide or pramlintide) is also being used.

Each day of the week, test your blood sugar just before every meal; just before your afternoon snack; just before your evening snack or, if you don't eat an evening snack, just before going to bed; prior to exercise; and before driving. Also, one day a week, test your blood sugar one to two hours after breakfast; on another day of the week, test one to two hours after lunch; and on a third day, test one to two hours after dinner. The following is an example of how you might set up this schedule:

Sunday: Test upon waking; before lunch; before your afternoon snack; before dinner; before your evening snack or at bedtime; and before exercising or driving.

Monday: Test upon waking; one to two hours after breakfast; before lunch; before your afternoon snack; before dinner; before your evening snack or at bedtime; and before exercising or driving.

Tuesday: Test upon waking, before lunch, before your afternoon snack, before dinner, before your evening snack or at bedtime, and before exercising or driving.

Wednesday: Test upon waking; before lunch; one to two hours after lunch; before your afternoon snack; before dinner; before your evening snack or at bedtime; and before exercising or driving.

Thursday: Test upon waking; before lunch; before your afternoon snack; before dinner; before your evening snack or at bedtime; and before exercising or driving.

Friday: Test upon waking; before lunch; before your afternoon snack; before dinner; one to two hours after dinner; before your evening snack or at bedtime; and before exercising or driving.

Saturday: Test upon waking; before lunch; before your afternoon snack; before dinner; before your evening snack or at bedtime; and before exercising or driving.

The pre-meal tests are necessary because they allow you and your diabetes care team to evaluate the effectiveness of your insulin doses. The pre-driving and pre-exercise tests are for safety purposes. The post-meal tests help you and your team to determine the optimal timing of your insulin doses.

Recording & Analyzing Your Results

If a tree falls in the forest and nobody hears it, does it make a sound? Of course it does. But what's the point?

More than Just Numbers

In recent years, a number of researchers have questioned the value of home blood sugar monitoring for people with type 2 diabetes. In each of the studies, however, a key element was neglected—teaching people to interpret their own information. Virtually every qualified diabetes specialist recommends home blood sugar monitoring for their patients with diabetes, because they recognize the value of home testing; they realize that intelligent adjustments to treatment can be made (by patients and/or their diabetes care team) when the test results are analyzed on a regular basis.

The same can be said about blood sugar tests. If you test your blood sugar and record the readings but then don't do anything with the results, what's the point? To make your testing worthwhile, you need to review and learn from your results. By keeping organized and accurate records of your blood sugar tests *and* analyzing them on a regular basis, you can gain tremendous insight into your diabetes management program.

At its most basic, your record keeping system should include the date and time of every blood sugar test and the results you obtained from each one. As long as your blood sugar readings are consistently within your target ranges, it is not usually necessary to keep track of anything else. But if some of the readings are above or below target, it becomes necessary to figure out why. Was a high or low reading caused by the consumption of too much or too little food? The wrong type, dose, or timing of medication? An unusual amount of physical activity? Stress? Illness? Every time you use your records to make a sensible adjustment to your treatment regimen (whether in the type, amount, or timing of food, physical activity, or medication), your blood sugar control will get a little bit better.

If you need to figure out why your blood sugar levels are straying outside their target ranges, you will need to record other information in addition to your test results. The same is true if your treatment regimen calls for injecting insulin at mealtimes, an approach that requires you to account for meals and physical activity in determining the correct dose of insulin. In either situation, you will need to record the major factors that influence blood sugar levels, including:

- The type, dose, and timing of any medication (oral medication, noninsulin injection, and/or insulin)

- The grams of carbohydrate consumed in each meal and snack (carb counting will be explained in detail in Step 10)

- The type and length of exercise and other physical activities performed, such as housework, yard work, shopping, and extended walking

- Stresses that tend to affect blood sugar levels, such as illnesses, menstrual cycles, emotional events, and hypoglycemic episodes

Your log sheets need not be fancy. A ruled notebook with columns and headers penciled in by hand will work just fine.

Learning how to interpret your self-monitoring records is also essential. Otherwise, your records are nothing more than pieces of paper covered with numbers and little spots of blood. To get the most from your record keeping, it helps to organize the information so it will be easy to analyze. One way is to line up several days' data in columns so that you can detect blood sugar patterns that occur at particular times of day. If you notice that your blood sugar levels are consistently high or low at a certain point each day, it is easy to make the right kind of adjustment to bring it back in line.

To see how this works, consider the table on page 91, which shows two weeks of blood sugar test results for Glenn Glucose. Glenn has type 2 diabetes and is currently taking no insulin or other medication for her diabetes. Her target ranges are:

Fasting (before breakfast): 70–100

Before other meals: 70–120

After meals: <140

	Before Breakfast	After Breakfast	Before Lunch	After Lunch	Before Dinner	After Dinner
Mon 3/1	95	166				
Wed 3/3			87	144		
Fri 3/5					77	158
Sun 3/7	99	190				
Tue 3/9			80	133		
Thu 3/11					100	202
Sat 3/13	81	175				

Notice how Glenn's pre-meal blood sugars are consistently near normal, but her after-meal readings are generally above her target range. It looks as though Glenn needs to work on managing her post-meal blood sugar, possibly through reduced carb intake at meals, some physical activity after meals, or the addition of a mealtime medication.

Now consider the results shown on page 93 for Greta Carbo. Greta is taking long-acting insulin once a day and oral diabetes medication at each meal. Her target ranges are:

Fasting (before breakfast): 70–120

Before other meals: 70–140

After meals: <160

Greta's pre- and post-meal blood sugars are all pretty close to her targets, except for her level first thing in the morning. Greta's dose of long-acting insulin likely needs to be increased, or she needs to reduce her late-night snacking. When you first begin testing, recording, and analyzing your own blood sugar levels, you should review your readings every couple of weeks. If they are fairly stable and within their target ranges, then monthly record reviews should be enough. But if you detect a pattern of readings that are out of range (above or below), bring them to the attention of your diabetes care team. Working with your team, you should be able to develop an effective solution for any

	Before Breakfast	After Breakfast	Before Lunch	After Lunch	Before Dinner	After Dinner	Bedtime
Mon 3/1	188	131					
Tue 3/2			102	122			
Wed 3/3					87	128	104
Thu 3/4	211	135					
Fri 3/5			110	114			
Sat 3/6					85	99	98

control problem. And as your experience grows, there will likely come a time when you will be able to determine for yourself what minor adjustments to make in your treatment regimen to bring any errant levels back where they belong. (But even then, you'll need regular check-ins with your diabetes care team.)

The Latest Advance in Blood Sugar Monitoring

The newest wave in diabetes management technology is **continuous glucose monitoring (CGM)**. Several systems are now available that provide blood sugar readings every couple of minutes and emit warnings when the sugar level is heading for a high or low. These systems use a sensor, a thin metallic filament inserted just below the skin, to detect sugar in the fluid between fat cells. They come with a spring-loaded device that makes inserting the sensor quick and relatively painless. The information from the sensor is transmitted via radio signals to a receiver that looks like a cell phone. The receiver displays charts, graphs, and an estimate of the current blood sugar level. The transmitter and receiver are reusable, although the sensor filament must be replaced every 5 to 15 days, depending on the specific system and the body's ability to tolerate the filament.

CGM devices are generally accurate to within about 15 percent of most finger-stick readings. They generate line graphs that depict sugar levels over the past several hours, allowing the user to detect trends and predict where blood sugar is headed. They use either vibration or a beeping noise to alert the wearer to impending high and low blood sugar levels. And computer or Web-based programs allow for detailed analysis of blood sugar levels over longer intervals of time.

Comparing finger-stick blood sugar testing to CGM is like comparing a photograph to a movie. CGM shows change and movement. It illustrates how virtually everything in daily life influences blood sugar levels. Used just once or twice, CGM can offer insight into the effectiveness of an individual's current diabetes management program. Worn on an ongoing basis, CGM makes it easier to keep blood sugars in range on a consistent basis with less risk of experiencing dangerous highs or lows.

Of course, CGM does have its drawbacks. It can be costly, and many health insurance plans resist covering it for people with type 2 diabetes. A CGM system requires some maintenance and technical know-how, and it's not always the most accurate testing method. It also still requires the user to enter the results from periodic finger-stick readings for calibration purposes. But if CGM sounds interesting to you, don't hesitate to talk to your diabetes care team to gather more information about it. Remember your attitude commitment: Don't let anything get between you and great control of your diabetes!

STEP 7:
Prepare to Unleash Your Lifestyle Tools

You may assume tight control relies on medication. Surprise! Three powerful and essential lifestyle tools may be all you need to successfully manage diabetes.

I F YOUR BLOOD sugar monitoring shows that your levels are out of control, it's time to use your lifestyle to bring them back in line. If that sounds like it's going to be anything but easy, the following true story might help change your view.

On the news the other day was a report about a man who was ticketed and arrested for driving illegally in a highway's HOV (high occupancy vehicle) lane. Such lanes are meant to encourage carpooling during high-traffic periods and are reserved, during those times, for cars carrying at least two people. The premise is simple: Go a little out of your way to find someone with whom you can share the drive, and you get to cruise past the usual congestion. Sounds fair, doesn't it?

Well, not to the guy who was arrested. Rather than finding someone to carpool with, he went to the trouble of producing an elaborate human-looking mannequin to put in the passenger seat. It was sad and comical at the same time. He described the painstaking process he went through to make the mannequin look as realistic as possible. The time and expense he put in were astronomical. Yet all they got him were a huge fine and a suspended license. And in a touch of poetic justice, he now has no choice but to find someone to give him rides!

All this brings us to our next lesson on the easy path to diabetes control: Trying to avoid managing your blood sugar can make life harder and less pleasant, as you struggle with the fatigue, discomforts, and disorders caused by poor control. Unleashing the lifestyle tools at your disposal, on the other hand, can make living in control far easier and make life itself more enjoyable.

Easy Diabetes Control Secret #7:

Sometimes it's easier to simply *do* the right things than it is to *avoid* doing them.

In the three steps that follow, we will focus on the "big three" lifestyle tools—physical activity, stress management, and proper eating—all three of which contribute to weight loss. Why does weight loss matter? Extra body fat robs insulin of much of its ability to lower blood sugar levels. Fat cells actually secrete hormones that cause insulin resistance throughout the body. The more overweight you are, the more insulin you will have to make or inject to control your blood sugar. But insulin also increases appetite and promotes more fat storage, making the insulin in your blood even less effective at pushing sugar into cells.

Your lifestyle tools, and the weight loss they often cause, can halt this dangerous downward spiral and help you bring your blood sugar levels under good control.

As you prepare to unleash those lifestyle tools, you'd be wise to enlist the help of professionals, at least at the start, to ensure you are making adjustments that are safe, effective, and appropriate for your specific condition(s), needs, and preferences. So if you haven't already, you should stock your diabetes care team with:

- An endocrinologist, who is a physician specially trained to treat people with hormone-related disorders such as diabetes, or an internist or general practitioner with extensive experience in treating people with diabetes

- An ophthalmologist (eye doctor), a dentist, and a podiatrist (foot doctor) experienced in treating the specific problems associated with diabetes in their respective fields

- A certified diabetes educator (CDE), who is a health professional (often a nurse, registered dietitian, exercise physiologist, or pharmacist, for example) with additional training in helping people with diabetes to manage their disease on a day-to-day basis

- A registered dietitian who has experience in helping people with type 2 diabetes to create and adopt a personalized meal plan and make food choices that will improve blood sugar control

- An exercise physiologist who has set up suitable exercise programs for other people with diabetes and worked with them to ensure they are executing the movements and activities safely and effectively

- A therapist, social worker, or other mental health counselor who understands the needs, concerns, and challenges of people living with a chronic disease such as diabetes

Your personal physician may be able to refer you to suitable candidates for these open spots on your diabetes care team. A family member or friend with diabetes may also have suggestions. You can also check the Web sites of various health and professional organizations; several have search functions that can provide you with the names of qualified members in your area (see the box Wanted: Expert Help on the following page).

Working together, you and your team of diabetes care professionals will be able to make the most of the lifestyle tools that are described in the upcoming steps so that you will not only be able to finally get control of your blood sugar but you will be able to keep it under control over the long term.

Wanted: Expert Help

You can visit the Web sites of the organizations listed below to locate health professionals in your area who can assist you in properly managing your diabetes.

American Academy of Ophthalmology
www.aao.org

American Association of Clinical Endocrinologists (AACE)
www.aace.com

American Association of Diabetes Educators (AADE)
www.diabeteseducator.org

American Dental Association (ADA)
www.ada.org

American Dietetic Association (ADA)
www.eatright.org

American Podiatric Medical Association (APMA)
www.apma.org

American Society of Exercise Physiologists (ASEP)
www.asep.org

STEP 8:
Get Moving

Physical activity can take you where you want to go in terms of blood sugar control, weight loss, and a lower risk of diabetic complications. It can even prevent diabetes from developing in the first place.

RECENTLY, ONE OF my clients, Betty, made an amazing discovery. "Gary, you won't believe this, but every time I go to the mall, my blood sugar comes down. And the more I spend, the more it drops!"

I didn't have the heart to tell her it wasn't the spending that was lowering her blood sugar. It was all the walking: Covering both levels of the mall meant more than a mile of walking. The more stores she explored, the more walking she did. And the more she bought, the more she wound up carrying. In other words, the more she worked her muscles, the more her blood sugar dropped.

You may not think of a brisk walk, housework, or washing the car as medicine for treating your diabetes, but it is. In fact, physical activity will not only help you better manage your diabetes; it will help treat, delay, or even prevent many of the long-term complications associated with diabetes.

Dress Your Feet for Success

Good athletic shoes are a must for nearly all types of cardiovascular, or aerobic, exercise. Today, sneakers are made differently for different types of activities. Most walking, running, or cross-training shoes will serve your purposes well. Be sure they're comfortable from the time you put them on; there should be no "break-in period" required. Shop for shoes in the evening, if possible, since feet tend to swell as the day progresses. Wear the socks you plan to have on during exercise, and try on both shoes to ensure they both fit properly. There should be at least half-inch of space, but not much more, between the tip of your big toe (or the second toe, if it is the longest) and the inside front of the shoe.

People with diabetes are at high risk for heart disease, high blood pressure, infection, elevated cholesterol, depression, and increased stress. Physical activity is a proven way to combat all of these conditions and burn extra calories, as well—an important benefit for those trying to lose weight.

As Betty discovered, physical activity is also a potent tool for lowering blood sugar, because it improves the way insulin works.

Imagine insulin as a key that opens cell doors, allowing sugar to float inside and be used for energy. Now, imagine the cells suddenly need more energy. The limited number of doors won't allow extra sugar to get in fast enough, so the sugar begins to back up outside the cells.

One solution would be to create more doors—and that's what physical activity does. When you engage in physical activity, your body temporarily creates more doors, allowing extra sugar to flow from the blood into the cells. After you've been inactive for a few hours, though, those new doors get sealed up again. But that's not the end of the story.

As discussed earlier, insulin resistance is an underlying cause of type 2 diabetes. The opposite of insulin resistance is **insulin sensitivity**, a state in which the body's cells are highly receptive to insulin. When the cells are more insulin sensitive, the pancreas doesn't need to make nearly as much insulin to keep the blood sugar in a normal range.

For people with type 2 diabetes, it is possible to improve insulin sensitivity *permanently* by losing weight and keeping it off, and physical activity can help with that. By being more physically active, many people with type 2 can increase their insulin sensitivity enough that they no longer need insulin injections or diabetes pills. In fact, it is possible to *prevent* diabetes through physical activity. The more calories a person burns per week exercising, the lower their risk of developing type 2 diabetes!

Physical activity also produces chemical messengers called **endorphins** that help relieve anxiety and pain and create a sense of euphoria. They also suppress the appetite in most people.

Enjoy the Magic of Movement

You may have noticed we haven't mentioned *exercise* even once. That's because physical activity need not include the kind of intense, sweat- and pain-inducing torture you may equate with exercise. Physical activity includes any form of purposeful movement that feels good. It should be safe and inexpensive (or free).

Being physically active every day is as much a state of mind as it is a state of being. Remember those "attitude" statements we made earlier? It's time to make one for physical activity, such as "I am not lazy. I am an active person, and I like to move."

The trouble is, today's society encourages us to be lazy. Our ancestors used to hunt, fish, build, clean, and walk just about all the time. Today, we hardly have to do anything for ourselves. I was at a store the other day and noticed that the doors open themselves, the escalators move us between floors, and even the soap and paper towels in the restroom come out on their own. These days, we actually have to go out of our way just to move!

For many people with blood sugar problems, the simple act of walking may be enough to start setting things right. Well, *that*, and a bit of motivation. To increase motivation, a **pedometer** can work wonders. This small device clips onto your waistband and tracks the number of times your hips shift position each day. It counts every time you get up, sit down, turn, jump, and step. It also reminds you that movement is good. Research has shown that people who wear pedometers and check them periodically throughout the day are motivated to walk and move more.

You should be able to find a basic pedometer for $10 to $20. It need not track anything other than the number of steps you take in a day. At the start, wear the pedometer around for a couple of days without changing your normal routine, just to see how many steps you currently average per day. Then aim to add a couple thousand more, and work toward meeting that goal. If you can work your way up to 10,000 steps or more per day, you will almost certainly be burning enough calories to improve your sensitivity to insulin.

Here are some ways you can increase your daily step count:

- Use a cordless phone, and walk while talking.

- When meeting friends, walk and talk instead of just sitting.

- Use stairs instead of elevators and escalators, particularly when going only one or two levels.

Keep It Simple

Pedometers can be found at most department stores and sporting goods stores. Look for one that isn't too complicated. All you need it to do is count your steps, not estimate distance or calories burned or read your mood like one of those rings from the '70s. As long as it has a button that lets you reset it each day, it should suit your needs.

- For nearby errands, leave the car in the garage and walk.

- Choose the farthest possible parking spot from the entrance at shopping centers and office buildings.

- Walk down every aisle in the grocery store, even if you only need a few things (and only if you can restrain yourself from buying snacks and sweets that you don't need).

- Adopt a dog and walk it two or three times a day.

- Get a treadmill and walk on it slowly while watching TV.

- Do your own yard work and housework. (Gardening will net you 70 to 80 steps per minute, and vacuuming will rack up more than 100!)

Stroll Your Way to Success

For a 200-pound person, walking at a slow pace burns about 300 calories per hour. While you're enjoying your favorite television shows, walk on a treadmill or even walk in place as you watch, and you'll see yourself get smaller!

- Instead of going out to movies or shows, do something active like dancing, bowling, or playing miniature golf. You can rack up 90 to 100 steps per minute while dancing!

- Hide the TV remote and get up to change channels.

- Take up an active hobby, like woodworking, sculpting, or bird-watching.

• Practice yoga, pilates, tai chi, or some other form of relaxing movement. Virtually every health club, YMCA, and adult education program offers classes that teach such activities. Many hospitals do, as well.

To make daily activity more fun, try an idea from one of my clients: For every 2,000 steps you accumulate on the pedometer, credit yourself one mile. Tack up a big state or regional map, and gradually move a pushpin toward a specific destination based on the number of miles you walk each day. Once the pushpin reaches the destination on the map, take a relaxing day trip there. You could use this approach as an excuse to visit family, friends, or any place you want to explore.

Make a Place for Exercise

Daily movement can certainly do a lot for you. But it can't do everything. To improve your cardiovascular (heart and blood vessel) fitness and make a serious attempt at weight loss, you'll need to perform physical activities that are a bit more challenging as well. You'll need to **exercise**. To qualify as exercise, an activity needs to engage large muscles in repetitive movement and raise your heart rate for an extended period of time.

The exercise activity you choose should be based on what you like to do, what you have access to, and what will be safe and

107

reasonable given your current health, abilities, and schedule. Be sure that you check with your doctor before starting any form of exercise, especially if you haven't been active recently.

Besides deciding on a type of exercise, you also need to consider when you will exercise, for how long, how often, and how intensely. If you have an exercise physiologist on your diabetes care team, you can work together to devise an effective, challenging, and safe exercise program that evolves as your fitness increases; the information in this step can facilitate your discussions. If you don't have access to such a professional, you can use the ideas that follow to design your own exercise program.

WHAT TO DO

Generally speaking, low-impact aerobic exercises are best, especially if you haven't exercised regularly in a long time. These are activities that don't involve a lot of jumping, pounding, or hitting anything with a lot of force (which can damage muscles, bones, and joints). Examples include swimming, cycling, "power walking," hiking, rowing, stair climbing, using an elliptical trainer, low-impact aerobics or water exercise, and dancing.

If your fitness level allows, however, you can include various court sports (tennis, basketball, racquetball, or squash, for example) as well as higher-impact activities (such as running, jumping rope, boxing, or martial arts). Weight lifting (strength training) also has its place in an exercise program and will be discussed in detail a bit later.

Even those who have problems with their lower extremities can engage in regular exercise. This includes anyone with very poor circulation or loss of nerve sensation in the legs or feet, as well as those with injuries, infections, or problems with balance. If you are in one of these categories, non-weight-bearing exercises are for you. These are activities in which you are not supporting your full body weight, such as stationary cycling, water exercise, upper-body weight lifting, armchair aerobics, or pedaling an arm ergometer (it's like a bicycle for your arms).

It's best to choose a variety of exercise activities, preferably ones that challenge different body parts. This is called **cross-training**. Cross-training helps you develop well-rounded fitness and prevents soreness from overuse of the same muscles and joints. Having choices also helps when you can't follow your usual routine due to injury, extreme weather, or travel. And it busts boredom, which can trump your best exercise intentions.

WHEN TO DO IT

When choosing a time of day to exercise, the first priority should be convenience. For long-term success, select a time of day that is conducive to your schedule and your lifestyle. That said, you may want to take advantage of the immediate blood-sugar-lowering effect of exercise and do it soon after eating a meal. For those who take insulin at each meal and want to lose weight, exercising after meals is optimal because you can cut back on your mealtime insulin dose and not have to worry about eating extra food just before exercising to ward off hypoglycemia. One major exception to the exercise-after-eating plan is the person who has been diagnosed with heart disease. A weak heart may be overstressed when exercise is performed too soon after eating. For such individuals, it's best to wait a couple hours after a meal before exercising.

Consistency is worth considering as well. Exercising at about the same time each day is best for improving blood sugar control and for sticking with an exercise program long-term. Because exercise can make your muscles more sensitive to insulin for several hours following the activity, exercising at the same time each day can help prevent unexpected peaks and valleys in your blood sugar levels. But if you need to vary the times of your workouts because of other commitments, that's perfectly fine; just be prepared to make adjustments to your insulin or medication as needed (which we'll discuss at the end of this step).

HOW OFTEN

Exercise is almost like medicine for people with diabetes in that it changes the way the body uses insulin. You wouldn't take your medicine only a few days a week, so you shouldn't exercise only a few days a week. Enjoy your exercise just about every day of the year. The more days you exercise, the better.

If you are completely new to exercise, it's okay to start with just a few days per week. But set your sights higher. Build up to five, six, or seven days a week as quickly as your body allows. I personally feel that it is fine to take a day off once in a while. Everyone needs a break or has an important commitment that gets in the way of exercise now and then. Beyond those rare exceptions, though, each day should include some form of exercise.

HOW INTENSELY

Forget "no pain, no gain." Pain means you're overdoing it or doing something improperly. Exercise should feel *good*. If it doesn't, ease up.

Moderate intensity is what you want to aim for. That means not too easy, not too hard—just right smack in the middle. There are three different methods you can use to judge whether you're in the middle: your heart rate (pulse), your rating of perceived exertion, and the "talk test."

You can take your pulse either at your wrist or, if you don't press too hard, on the side of your Adam's apple. (Check your pulse as you continue the activity, if possible; otherwise, stop only long enough to count the heartbeats.) Counting your pulse for ten seconds will let you know if you are above, below, or within what is called your **target heart-rate range** during exercise. (Note that these ranges apply only to those who are *not* taking any medication that limits heart rate, such as beta blockers for high blood pressure; if you take any such medication, ask your doctor or exercise physiologist what your target range should be.) If your pulse count during exercise is above the range listed in the table below, slow down. If it is below, speed up a bit. Keep in mind that even if you maintain the same intensity, your pulse rate may go up during the course of a workout as you begin to fatigue, so check your pulse every five or ten minutes throughout your workout to ensure you're still in your target range.

Your Age	Ten-Second Target Heart-Rate Range During Exercise
20–29	20–26
30–39	19–25
40–49	18–23
50–59	17–22
60–69	16–21
70–79	15–19
80+	14–18

Your second option for measuring intensity is a bit less scientific but nonetheless effective. It is called the **Rating of Perceived Exertion** scale, or **RPE.** RPE relies simply on your own evaluation of how hard you are working at any given moment. Aim to keep your intensity in the "target zone" shown in the table below.

RPE Zone	Description
0	Complete rest
1	Very, very easy
2	Very easy
3	Easy
4	Moderately easy
5	Moderate
6	Moderately hard
7	Hard
8	Very hard
9	Very, very hard
10	Absolute maximal effort

}**TARGET ZONE** (zones 4–6)

The third way to track your intensity—the **talk test**—is very unscientific but practical all the same. It relies on this simple guideline: You should be able to hold a conversation, but not be able to sing, when exercising at the right intensity. If you're having difficulty carrying on a light conversation, you're working too hard. If you can belt out a few verses of your favorite song, you need to increase the intensity. What could be simpler?

FOR HOW LONG

If you have not exercised for many years (or ever), it is fine to start out at an easy pace for just a few minutes at a time and then gradually build up the length of your exercise sessions by adding one minute each time you exercise. You should aim to reach at least 30 minutes of continuous exercise. If you can go longer and you want to lose weight a little bit quicker, gradually build up to one 60-minute exercise session or two 30-minute exercise sessions each day.

Once you have reached the desired workout length, start to slowly increase your speed or intensity. This will keep you within your target range as your fitness level improves, and it will keep your workouts challenging and stimulating.

Your 30 to 60 minutes of exercise per day should include a few minutes of warm-up and cool-down time spent in a slow, easy version of your chosen exercise. If you plan to walk briskly for exercise, for example, start and finish your workout with three to five minutes of casual walking. This allows your heart rate to adjust gradually and safely as you begin and end your workout.

Jump-Start Your Metabolism

You can burn plenty of additional calories each day by exercising and increasing your overall level of physical activity. But we're going to let you in on a little secret: There's a way you can burn extra calories when you're not lifting a finger. It involves something called your basal metabolic rate. Your basal metabolic rate refers to the calories your body burns just to keep your heart beating, lungs breathing, eyes blinking...in other words, just to keep you alive. This calorie expenditure is like the interest you earn on a bank account: It's essentially something you get for doing nothing but being there.

Fat is metabolically stagnant. Fat cells require virtually no calories to stay alive. Muscle, on the other hand, is very active metabolically. Muscle cells chew through a lot of calories even when they aren't moving. The more muscle you have, the higher your basal metabolism and the more calories your body burns all the time—even when you're resting. Adding muscle is like turning a savings account that pays 3 percent interest into a high-yield account that earns 8 percent.

Cardiovascular, or aerobic, exercise will tone your muscles, strengthen your heart, improve blood flow throughout your body, and help improve your blood sugar levels. But it won't necessarily do much to make your muscles bigger (if you're a man) or denser

115

(if you're a woman). "Adding muscle" requires **strength training,** also known as weight lifting. Strength training involves moderate to high exertion for short periods of time. When a muscle is worked to near (but not quite) exhaustion, the muscle becomes stronger and more efficient. Stronger and more efficient muscles burn more calories every minute of the day, whether you are actively working them or not, and they can help you achieve your weight loss goals more quickly.

If your diabetes care team includes an exercise physiologist, he or she can work with you to design and implement a strength-training routine to suit your needs and abilities. If you have access to a health club, ask a member of the fitness staff to demonstrate how to use the various machines properly. If you plan to lift weights on your own, you can use ordinary household objects for weights: Cans, bottles, rocks, rolls of coins, or anything else that is small, dense, and easy to grip. You'll find sample muscle-building exercises you can perform with hand weights at the back of the book, and you'll find information on designing a strengthening routine below.

As with any form of exercise, when you start lifting weights, it is best to start very slow and easy; otherwise, you could wind up very sore and discouraged afterward. For the first week, you should use a comfortable weight to perform just one set of ten repetitions (reps) of each weight-lifting exercise. The second week, increase to two sets with a pause in between. The third week, do three sets with a pause between each. Once you can do three sets of ten reps, you're ready to start increasing your reps. Once you can perform three sets of 15 reps using proper technique, increase the weight but return to three sets of ten. Once again work up to doing three sets of 15 reps using proper form, and then increase the weight again. Continue this cycle of gradually increasing the reps and the weight until you reach a plateau and find it difficult to increase the weight or do additional reps. Don't feel discouraged when you get to this point; everyone reaches a plateau. Just work on perfecting your technique.

You will progress faster and/or further or reach a plateau sooner on some exercises than you do on others. It helps to track your weight-lifting progress by keeping a simple log or diary in a spiral-bound notebook or binder. For each exercise in your routine, write down the date, the weight you used, and the number of sets and reps you were able to perform before your technique failed (in other words, before you no longer had the strength to execute the exercise properly) or you simply couldn't lift the weight any more. The next time you do the exercise, check this record to see how far you got with it the last time, and try to take it a step further.

Here are a few pointers to help make your weight-lifting workouts safer and more effective:

1. **Warm up before lifting.** Walk or ride a stationary bike for a few minutes before you begin a round of weight-lifting, and mimic each exercise (minus the weight) before performing it.

2. **Lift in the proper order.** Start with exercises that work the big muscles in the chest, back, thighs, and shoulders, and end with lifts that train the smaller muscles of the arms and lower legs. When going through your lifting routine, try to alternate between exercises that work your arms and shoulders, those that strengthen your abdomen and lower back, and those that focus on your buttocks and legs.

3. **Never hold your breath when lifting weight.** This can cause a dangerous rise in blood pressure. Blow air out when you raise the weight, and inhale as you lower it.

4. **Skip a day between weight-lifting workouts.** This gives your muscles time to recover and become stronger.

5. **When increasing weight, do so in very small increments.** For example, going from lifting five pounds to ten pounds represents a 100-percent increase in weight, and that's too much of a jump. Go, instead, from lifting five pounds to six or seven (maybe 7.5) pounds.

6. **Do not proceed until your technique is perfect.** Be sure you can maintain the proper form for every single rep

before you increase the weight or the number of reps. If you struggle with the last couple reps, stay where you are until you can do them all properly.

7. **Lift and lower weight using slow, controlled movements.**
Slow lifts produce the best results.

Besides strength training, another way you can raise your metabolism is by doing something called **interval training**. In interval training, you perform cardiovascular exercise at alternating high and low intensities. For example, you could walk for several minutes and then jog or sprint for a couple of minutes, then return to walking for several minutes, then back to jogging for two minutes, and so on, repeating the sequence several times throughout your workout. As your conditioning improves, you can shorten your low-intensity intervals and lengthen your high-intensity intervals to keep your workouts challenging.

Interval training has been shown to improve stamina and produce a higher metabolic rate.

How's This for Motivation?

The 2006–07 winner of the Mr. Universe contest is a competitive power lifter and bodybuilder named Doug Burns. Doug was diagnosed with diabetes at age 7. And when he started lifting weights as a teen, he had nothing more than scrap metal to use as weights. Talk about not letting anything hold you back!

Put It All Together

Now you know that movement of all kinds is vital to controlling blood sugar and preventing or treating diabetes. You know you need to increase your level of physical activity every day in every way you can. And you know you need to schedule both cardiovascular and strength-training workouts into your regular routine. So what would such a workout plan look like? Below is an example of a workout plan that I put together for a client of mine named Jackie.

JACKIE'S WORKOUT PLAN

Type(s) of Exercise	Walk outdoors (ride stationary bike in bad weather) Use hand weights
When?	Before breakfast (workdays) After breakfast (days off)
How Often?	Walk or bike: 4 times per week (Sat, Sun, 2 weekdays) Weights: 2 times per week (weekdays)
How Intensely?	Walk or bike: Easy while building up to 40 minutes; then moderate Weights: 3 sets of 10; build up to 3 sets of 15
For How Long?	Walk or bike: Start with 10 minutes; add 1 minute each day, up to 40 minutes.

It can seem a bit overwhelming to think of anything (including exercise) as a lifelong commitment, so it's best to focus on manageable chunks. In Jackie's case, she committed to following her workout program one week at a time. At the start of each week, she would simply renew her commitment. That approach seems to have worked well: I designed the workout plan for her in 1998, and Jackie is *still* sticking with it.

Adjust for Physical Activity

Sometimes, the truth hurts. One truism facing people with diabetes is this: The more insulin you take (or the more insulin your body makes), the harder it is to burn fat and lose weight. But the opposite is also true: The less insulin you take (or make), the easier it is for your body to burn fat and lose weight. That's why it's so important to take advantage of any opportunity that allows you to cut back on your insulin levels without harming your blood sugar control.

Physical activity creates just such an opportunity. Because physical activity makes your insulin work far more effectively, you simply don't need as much of it. In fact, if you inject insulin or use a medication that stimulates your pancreas to make more insulin, and you *don't* reduce your medication dose to account for physical activity, you could wind up with hypoglycemia (low blood sugar).

Medications that *Can* Cause Hypoglycemia	Medications that *Do Not* Cause Hypoglycemia
• **Insulin** (all forms) • **Sulfonylureas** (glipizide, glyburide) • **Meglitinides** (Prandin, Starlix) • **Combination Medications** that contain any of the above	• **Metformin** (Glucophage) • **Acarbose** (Precose) • **Thiazoladinediones** (Actos, Avandia) • **DPP4 Inhibitors** (Januvia) • **Incretin Mimetics** (Byetta, Symlin)

If you do not use a medication that can cause hypoglycemia, you do not need to worry about snacking, reducing your medication dose, or doing anything else before or during your workouts to adjust for exercise. If you do use insulin or a drug that increases your body's insulin production, however, you will need to make some commonsense adjustments that will help you both prevent low blood sugar and lose weight faster; they are discussed below. Just be sure to check with your diabetes care team before making any of your own dosage adjustments.

If you take rapid-acting insulin at mealtimes or use a pre-mixed formulation that contains rapid-acting insulin, it is a good idea to reduce your insulin dose at the meal prior to your physical activity. The chart at the top of the next page should help.

	Short duration (15–30 minutes)	**Moderate** duration (31–60 minutes)	**Long** duration (1–2 hours)
Low intensity (relatively easy)	10% reduction	25% reduction	33% reduction
Moderate intensity	25% reduction	33% reduction	50% reduction
High intensity (very challenging)	33% reduction	50% reduction	67% reduction

For example, if you plan to garden for two hours after lunch and would normally take 10 units of rapid-acting insulin, you should lower the dose by 33 percent, to roughly 7 units. If you plan a brisk, 45-minute swim after lunch and normally take 8 units of insulin, you should reduce your dose by 50 percent, to 4 units.

For activities of longer duration, such as day hikes or several hours of yard work, you may need to reduce your long-acting insulin (NPH, Lantus, or Levemir). It is reasonable to reduce the dose of long-acting insulin by 25 percent either the night before or the morning of such an action-packed day.

Also, you should be prepared for the possibility of a delayed blood sugar drop, particularly after a long or very intense workout. There are two reasons such a drop can occur. The muscle cells' enhanced sensitivity to insulin, which normally occurs after activity, is prolonged when the exercise itself is prolonged. And the muscle cells need to replenish their own energy stores following such exhaustive exercise. If you tend to experience a drop in blood sugar several hours after heavy exercise, you can prevent it by lowering your long-acting and rapid-acting insulin by 25 percent following the workout or by having an extra snack prior to the time the drop in blood sugar tends to occur. Ideally, the snack should contain slowly digesting carbohydrates, such as whole fruit, milk, yogurt, or peanut butter.

If you take insulin or a medication that can cause hypoglycemia, there are certain situations in which you will need to consume extra food to prevent hypoglycemia. One example is when you will be exercising before or between meals. The size of the snack you'll need will depend on the duration and intensity of your workout. The harder and longer your muscles will be working, the more carbohydrate you will need to maintain your blood sugar level. The amount is also based on your body size: The bigger you are, the more fuel you will burn while exercising, and the more carbohydrate you will need.

There is no way of knowing *exactly* how much carbohydrate you will need, but the table on the next page should provide a safe starting point. Select the intensity level at which you plan to exercise, and follow that row until it intersects with the weight closest to your own. There you will find a range of numbers. If you weigh roughly the amount listed at the top of the column, select an amount of carbohydrate grams in the middle of the range given. If you weigh less than the amount at the top, opt for a number of grams closer to the lower end of the given range. And if you weigh more than the amount listed at the top, choose a number of grams at the higher end of the given range.

Keep in mind that the range of numbers given in the chart represents the grams of carbohydrate that you will need *per hour* of activity. If you'll be exercising for half an hour, eat half the listed amount before you begin the activity. If you'll be exercising for two hours, take the entire amount at the start of each hour.

Carbohydrate Needed Per **60 Minutes** of Physical Activity					
	100 lbs	150 lbs	200 lbs	250 lbs	300 lbs
Low Intensity	10–16g	15–25g	20–32g	25–40g	30–45g
Moderate Intensity	20–26g	30–40g	40–52g	50–65g	60–75g
High Intensity	30–36g	45–55g	60–72g	75–90g	90–110g

To confirm that you have chosen the optimal size and frequency for your snacks, test your blood sugar before and after the activity. If it has held steady, you chose the right amount. If it has gone up, you will need to cut back on the grams of carbohydrate you eat before (or at the start of each hour of) your next exercise session. And if your blood sugar has dropped, you will need to eat more carbohydrate before (or at the start of each hour of) your next workout or you will need to eat more frequently during your exercise session the next time.

If you take a medication other than insulin that can cause hypoglycemia, it is usually recommended that you take your usual dose for your first couple of exercise sessions and see what happens. If your blood sugar drops below 80 mg/dl during or after exercise, be sure to alert your diabetes care team. You may need to reduce or eliminate the medication or switch to a medication that does not cause hypoglycemia. Check with your doctor before you make any medication changes, however.

Despite the precautions you take, hypoglycemia can still occur if you take insulin or a medication that stimulates your pancreas to release more insulin. If you fall into either category, therefore, you should always carry a source of simple sugar (such as glucose tablets, a sports drink, juice, or hard candy) and wear a medical alert bracelet or necklace (identifying you as a person with diabetes) whenever you exercise. Stop the activity and treat the low blood sugar as soon as you suspect it, and take a timeout of at least 15 to 20 minutes to allow the food to be absorbed. Wait until your blood sugar is a minimum of 90 mg/dl before continuing physical activity.

Oddly enough, physical activity can actually cause blood sugar to rise in certain circumstances, particularly at the onset of high-intensity, short-duration exercise. This is caused by a surge of the stress hormone adrenaline. If you detect such an increase, talk with your doctor about ways to offset or prevent it. Although high blood sugar can impair your performance during exercise, it is not necessarily dangerous to exercise when blood sugar levels are moderately elevated. If you experience high blood sugar during exercise, drink plenty of water during and after your workouts. If you experience very high blood sugar with exercise, alert your doctor and ask whether you should be checking your urine for ketones, which are acidic by-products produced when fat is metabolized. It is a good idea to check for ketones if your blood sugar is greater than 300 mg/dl. A positive ketone test could mean that you are deficient in insulin, and in that case, physical activity will probably make your blood sugar go much higher. Do not exercise if your urine contains ketones.

STEP 9:
Manage Stress

Your body releases more sugar into the blood when stressed, so if your aim is tighter control, relieving stress is important.

O NE NIGHT, I decided to stay up late and watch a scary movie about a mummy that came to life and started munching on unsuspecting tourists. After the locals fought back and the final mummy had been dispatched, I decided to check my blood sugar. It had gone up more than 100 points since the movie started, even though I hadn't eaten a thing. How could that happen? The answer can be found in a look at early humans.

In the Stone Age, things *were* pretty simple. There were no in-laws or tax forms or computer viruses to worry about. But there were hungry, human-eating animals with sharp claws and big teeth. The mere sight or sound of these creatures would give our early ancestors an adrenaline rush so powerful that they could outrun or out-wrestle just about any wild animal. This "fight or flight" reaction helped the first humans to survive.

We know now that an adrenaline rush increases the heart rate, dilates the pupils, tenses the muscles, causes sweating, stops digestion, and makes the liver release a jolt of sugar into the bloodstream for quick energy. All of these responses are very helpful when we're threatened with bodily harm. Unfortunately, our bodies can't tell the difference between a *physical* threat and an *emotional* threat, so our response to everyday mental stress and psychological pressure is very similar to the way we would respond if we were being chased by an animal. You certainly don't *need* your blood pressure, heart rate, and blood sugar to go up every time your computer screen flashes "Fatal Recovery Error." (Running away or fighting the machine won't help.) But it happens nonetheless. And it is what we call a **stress response.**

Emotional stresses such as fear, anxiety, anger, excitement, and tension cause the body to produce adrenaline and other stress hormones. These stress hormones, in turn, cause the liver to secrete extra sugar into the blood. They also increase insulin resistance. For people without diabetes, the stress-induced rise in blood sugar is followed by an increase in insulin secretion, so the blood sugar spike is modest and momentary. For people with diabetes, however, stress can cause blood sugar to rise quickly and stay high for quite a while.

We all have some degree of stress in our lives. The difference is that some people dwell on their stress and let it get to them more so than other people do.

You can't avoid stressful situations completely—nor would you want to, since even happy events cause emotional stress—but you can learn to contain and manage the common ones. To begin, it helps to list the people, places, and situations that typically cause stress for you. Once you've identified frequent stressors, examine them calmly and realistically to see if you can discern ways to avoid/prevent them, lessen their impact, or cope with them more effectively (without letting them hijack your thoughts and emotions or ruin your day). Then try some of the following suggestions for dealing with everyday stressors.

- Keep a sense of humor. Laughing is a tremendous way to let go of stress. When you laugh, your body produces natural painkillers and increases circulation. And just thinking about something funny can put stressful situations into proper perspective.

Say "Ohm"

Meditation, accompanied by slowly paced breathing, has the proven ability to calm and focus the mind, lower blood pressure, and put the body into a relaxed state. Practiced on a regular basis, it can be used to blunt the traditional stress response during difficult situations and to prepare ourselves for challenging events.

- If waiting in lines or traffic causes you stress, plan ahead with things to do while you wait.

- Find a temporary escape. Even though you should not "run away" from your problems, a temporary reprieve can be very helpful. Immerse yourself in music. Take a vacation. Visit nature. Or just pamper yourself with a massage, aromatherapy, or an old-fashioned bubble bath.

• Simplify your life. Overcommitment is a major source of stress for many people. Shop less, and spend well within your means. When it comes to committing your time and energy, learn the value of saying "No" sometimes.

• If overwork causes you stress, make to-do lists for yourself, prioritize tasks, and delegate whenever possible to help lessen your load. If your job is a major source of ongoing stress, it may be time to re-evaluate your position or career.

• Find a release valve. Some people benefit from writing down the causes of their stress and how it makes them feel. Simply getting it all down on paper may provide some relief. Others find comfort in talking things out with a friend or therapist. (Or you could try my wife's favorite stress reliever: hitting baseballs in a batting cage.)

• If people close to you cause you stress, don't try to change them. Try to understand why they act the way they do, and don't take their actions too personally.

• Run—or walk or pedal or swim—away from your stressors for a little while. Exercise removes us from our problems. It also improves blood flow to the brain, which may help us come up with creative solutions for them. Regular exercise also makes us feel more in control of our bodies and our lives, which in itself can weaken the stress response.

- Do volunteer work. Helping others and giving of yourself can give your spirits a real lift. It can also put your own issues in perspective and is a great way to refocus on things that are truly important in life.

- Sleep it off. Sleep deprivation can be a major source of physical and emotional stress and can lessen our ability to cope with other stressors. Invest in a comfortable bed and pillow. Avoid caffeine and heavy eating at night. Develop a bedtime routine that relaxes you and helps you to fall asleep.

- Practice progressive muscle relaxation. Tighten and release your muscles one group at a time, from face to toes, spending about ten seconds on each muscle group. This forces your muscles to relax. Simply knowing how your muscles feel when you are relaxed will make it easier for you to detect when you're feeling tense in response to stress.

If these techniques don't do the job, consider seeking professional help. Most mental health professionals are trained in helping clients deal effectively with stress. (A psychiatrist may also prescribe a temporary course of medication.) A mental health professional can also determine if clinical depression, which is very common in people with diabetes, is playing a role.

STEP 10:
Eat for Control

Understanding how your food choices affect your blood sugar is absolutely essential.

N o APPROACH TO tight control would be complete without a sound eating plan. As a wise doctor once told a group of patients, "Modern science has brought us some amazing medicines for treating diabetes. But the bottom line is this: You can still out-eat anything I prescribe for you."

There are three main factors you need to consider when making your food choices:

1. Carbohydrates, because they have the greatest immediate impact on your blood sugar level;

2. Glycemic index, because in many cases the *rate* at which you digest is just as important as *what* you digest;

3. Calories, because you need to balance your energy intake against your energy expenditure.

Understanding these factors and properly taking them into account when making food choices are central to bringing blood sugar under control.

Carbohydrates

Carbohydrates (carbs, for short) include simple sugars such as sucrose (table sugar), fructose (fruit sugar), lactose (milk sugar), and corn syrup, as well as complex carbs, better known as starches. You can think of a simple sugar as an individual railroad car and a starch as a bunch of cars hooked together to make a train. Most starches are composed of many sugar molecules linked together.

The carbs you eat are converted by your body into glucose, the sugar that circulates through your bloodstream to nourish your body's cells. Blood sugar is your body's primary fuel. To get the sugar out of your bloodstream and into your body's cells, your pancreas produces insulin. Consuming large amounts of carbohydrate places a heavy workload on the pancreas; so does eating carbs that digest very quickly, because the pancreas must pump out insulin at a furious rate to keep up with the sudden rush of sugar into the bloodstream. In people who are insulin resistant or who have a pancreas that has a hard time keeping up, there simply may not be enough insulin produced to keep the blood sugar level from going too high. Because carbs contain four calories per gram, consuming excessive amounts of carbohydrate will also contribute to weight gain, which makes the body's cells even more insulin resistant.

Foods Rich in Sugar (simple carbs)	Foods Rich in Starch (complex carbs)
Fruit	Potatoes
Fruit juice	Rice
Raisins/Dried fruit	Noodles/Pasta
Regular soda	Cereal
Punch	Oatmeal
Candy	Bread
Chocolate	Crackers
Cookies & Cakes	Bagels
Pies & Pastries	Pizza
Muffins	Tortillas
Milk	Pancakes
Ice cream	Waffles
Yogurt	Beans
Sports drinks	Corn
Table sugar	Pretzels
Honey	Chips
Syrup	Popcorn
Jelly	Beer

Now here's the statement that sends most people running to call that cousin who claims to know everything. *From the standpoint of blood sugar control, it doesn't matter if the carbs you eat are simple sugars or complex carbs (starches), because both will raise blood sugar by the same amount.* A cup of rice containing 50 grams of com-

Bagel or Donut?

They're both round, they both have a hole in the middle, and they both taste pretty good. But which is better in terms of your blood sugar? Believe it or not, two glazed donuts have fewer carbohydrates than does one typical bagel-shop bagel. And the bagel actually raises blood sugar faster than the donuts do. But don't get too excited. The donuts contain four to eight times as much fat as the bagel, and that's also an important consideration for people with type 2 diabetes, since excess body fat impairs blood sugar control. Instead, try an English muffin with a tablespoon of jam or a slice of toast with a tablespoon of peanut butter.

plex carbohydrate will raise the blood sugar just as much as a can of regular, sugar-sweetened soda that contains 50 grams of simple sugars will. And both will raise it pretty fast. In other words, when you're evaluating how a particular food will affect your blood sugar, don't be overly concerned about its *sugar content*; instead, focus on its *total carbohydrate content*.

How much carbohydrate should you eat? That depends on many things: How tall you are, how physically active you are, how much weight you need to lose, and other factors. To determine the precise amount of carbohydrate you should be having at each meal and snack, it is best to meet with a registered dietitian (R.D.) who is also a certified diabetes educator (C.D.E.) or has experience counseling people

REASONABLE DAILY CARBOHYDRATE INTAKE FOR PEOPLE WITH (OR AT RISK OF) TYPE 2 DIABETES:

	Short Stature		Medium Stature		Tall Stature	
	Male	Female	Male	Female	Male	Female
Fairly Inactive	120–140g	110–130g	140–160g	120–140g	180–210g	140–160g
Moderately Active	160–190g	130–160g	190–220g	140–170g	220–250g	160–190g
Very Active	180–220g	150–190g	220–260g	160–200g	250–300g	180–220g

with diabetes. (See Step 7 for information on adding a dietitian to your diabetes care team.) Most health insurance plans will cover all or part of the cost of meeting with a dietitian at least once. And even if they don't, it's still well worth the cost. (Remember your attitude adjustment: Don't let minor costs get in the way of taking care of yourself!)

Until you can meet with a dietitian and develop an individualized plan, you can use the general carbohydrate recommendations that follow to get started. First, you need to estimate how much carbohydrate you should have in a typical day. The amounts shown in the table on page 137 are slightly less than those generally recommended by the U.S. Department of Agriculture for most Americans and provide a reasonable starting range of intake—based on

No-Carb No-No

Everyone needs some carbohydrate in their diet. Carbs are the primary source of the glucose that cells use for energy, and the body easily turns carbs into blood sugar. If you consume no carbs, your body is forced to dismantle valuable protein (the stuff muscles are made of) for fuel, something it prefers not to do. In the absence of carbs, your body also begins breaking down fat for fuel, but the byproducts (called ketones) that result can, over time, throw off your body's acid-base balance and damage your liver and kidneys. Meanwhile, you are left vulnerable to bouts of lethargy and low blood sugar.

gender, height/body size, and activity level—for people who have or are at risk of type 2 diabetes.

For example, if you are a woman of medium height who is not very active physically, you should aim for a total of about 120 to 140 grams of carbohydrate per day. If you are a tall, moderately active man, aim for about 220 to 250 grams per day.

Once you have an idea of how much total carbohydrate to consume daily, you need to know how to distribute it throughout the day. After all, nobody expects you to consume 150 grams of carbohydrate in one sitting. It would not only be impractical; it would put too much strain on your body's ability to regulate blood sugar following a meal. Instead, divide your carbs among (at least) three meals and one or two snacks per day.

For example, if you have 160 grams of carbohydrate to "spend" for the day, you could have 30 grams for breakfast, 45 for lunch, 20 in an afternoon snack, 45 for dinner, and 20 in an evening snack. Remember that the goal is to keep your total carbohydrate intake within a reasonable range and avoid flooding your bloodstream with too much glucose at any one sitting.

CARBOHYDRATE COUNTING TECHNIQUES

Keeping your daily carbohydrate intake in a reasonable range is important for regaining control of your blood sugar levels, but it requires you to have a system for quantifying the amount of carbohydrate in the foods you eat—in other words, a technique for *carb counting*. By counting carbs, people in the early stages of type 2 diabetes can avoid overworking the pancreas. And for those in more advanced stages of diabetes, carb counting allows them to match insulin doses to the food being eaten. What follows are discussions of the primary carb counting methods.

1. Carb Exchanging

One of the most basic methods for counting carbs involves converting food types into grams of carbohydrate. It is based on the traditional, more complex diabetic "Exchange System," in which foods are grouped by their typical nutrient content. For example, one slice of bread counts as one "starch." A small apple is counted as one "fruit."

You may have heard people with diabetes say they get "three breads at breakfast, four at lunch, four at dinner, and two at bedtime." In this context, a "bread" may mean a slice of bread *or* a food similar in carbohydrate, fat, and protein

Exchange *This!*

The vast majority of diabetes experts these days prefer carb counting systems to the older "Exchange System," and with good reason. In the 1980s, a group of nurses was placed on an exchange meal plan for a week. Almost none of these medical professionals were able to follow it, citing the complexity, rigidity, and inaccuracy inherent in the system.

content to a slice of bread. A slice of bread has lots of carbs (15 grams per serving), with a small amount of protein and fat. The same can be said for a half cup spaghetti, three cups popcorn, or $\frac{1}{3}$ cup corn. In other words, three cups of popcorn can be "exchanged" for a slice of bread because it contains about the same carb count.

The same holds true for the other exchanges. Just like a typical piece of meat, a "meat" exchange has very few carbs, a lot of protein, and a moderate-to-high amount of fat.

The table on page 142 shows examples of foods in each exchange group and their approximate per-serving nutrient content:

Beyond the Scale

If you've chosen the healthy path to weight loss and have begun including daily exercise along with dietary changes, the bathroom scale may not reflect all the progress you're making, because you may be losing more fat than pounds. Many forms of exercise can help you to burn off pounds of unsightly, unhealthy body fat, but some can also add lean mass, or lean weight, by building toned, calorie-burning muscle and denser, stronger bones. So rather than using the scale alone to gauge your progress, you should also measure your chest, waist, and hips with a tape measure or ask a fitness professional to measure your body fat percentage. These additional measures will provide you with "hard" evidence that you're losing fat and building muscle.

Exchange Group	Carbohydrate	Protein	Fat
Bread: 1 slice bread; ¾ cup corn flakes; 6 saltine crackers; ½ cup noodles	Lots (15g)	Little (3g)	Little (1g)
Fruit: ½ cup orange juice; 1 small apple; ½ banana; 1 cup watermelon	Lots (15g)	None (0g)	None (0g)
Vegetable: ⅓ cup cooked carrots; ½ cup fresh peas; 1 cup spinach; ½ cup canned tomato	Little (5g)	Little (2g)	None (0g)
Milk: 1 cup milk or unsweetened yogurt	Moderate (12g)	Lots (8g)	Varies (1–8g)
Meat: 1 oz. meat, cheese, or cold cuts; 2 tbs. peanut butter	None (0g)	Lots (7g)	Varies (3–8g)
Fat: 1 tsp. butter; 1 strip bacon; 1 tsp. vegetable oil; 2 tbs. sour cream	None (0g)	None (0g)	Lots (5g)

The following list shows you how many grams of carbohydrate you get from a single selection in each exchange.

1 "Bread" Exchange	= 15 grams carb
1 "Fruit" Exchange	= 15 grams carb
1 "Milk" Exchange	= 12 grams carb
1 "Vegetable" Exchange	= 5 grams carb
1 "Meat" Exchange	= 0 grams carb
1 "Fat" Exchange	= 0 grams carb

To figure out how much carbohydrate you're having in a meal, add up the grams of carbohydrate you are getting from each exchange. A meal of two breads (2 × 15), two fruits (2 × 15), a milk (1 × 12), and three meats (3 × 0) supplies a total of 72 grams of carbohydrate. Just be sure your portions match the definition of a single serving in each food's exchange. For example, a small apple counts as a single "fruit" exchange, but if the apple you are eating is medium or large, it counts as 1½ or 2 "fruit" exchanges, so your carb calculation needs to reflect this. You'll find a more detailed exchange list at the back of this book.

2. Label Reading

When it comes to carb counting, food labels can be your best friend. The U.S. Food and Drug Administration (FDA) requires all packaged and processed foods to list pertinent nutrient information such as total grams of carbohydrate, grams of sugar, and grams of fiber in a single serving of the food. **Fiber** is a unique type of carbohydrate in that it passes through the body undigested and thus adds no calories and has little effect on blood sugar. Most foods contain little or no fiber, so for them, the total carbohydrate figure on the label can be used for carb counting. For foods that do contain fiber, you'll need to subtract the grams of fiber from the grams of total carbohydrate to arrive at the number of carbohydrate grams to use in carb counting.

Let's take a look at an example. The Nutrition Facts label shown here is for a food item that contains 29 grams of total carbohy-

Nutrition Facts

Serving Size ½ cup
Servings Per Container 8

Amount Per Serving

Calories 125   Calories from fat 18

% Daily Value*

Total Fat 2g	**4%**
Saturated Fat 0g	**0%**
Trans Fat 0g	**0%**
Cholesterol 0mg	**0%**
Sodium 120mg	**5%**
Total Carbohydrate 29g	**10%**
Dietary Fiber 3g	
Sugars 16g	
Protein 2g	

* Percent Daily Values are based on a 2,000 calorie diet.

drate per serving. The 16 grams of sugar are already included in the total carbohydrate figure, so there is no need to count them separately. A single serving also contains 3 grams of fiber, which you *do* need to subtract from the 29 grams of total carbohydrate, leaving you with 26 grams of digestible carbs to include in your carb count that day.

144

It's also important to be sure the amount you eat matches the serving size listed on the label. If your portion is smaller or larger

No Label? No Problem.

Nutrient labels make carb counting easy, but only if there's a label on every food you eat. Unpackaged foods, such as fresh fruits and vegetables, some baked goods, fast foods, and made-to-order foods, typically do not carry labels. For these, you need to refer to a printed or electronic nutrient guide that lists the serving size and the per-serving amounts of total carb, fiber, and calories for unlabeled foods.

Fortunately, you can access the U.S. Government's free nutrient database at http://www.nal.usda.gov/fnic/foodcomp/search/. You can use the Web site's search function to view the carb and calorie counts for specific serving sizes of thousands upon thousands of foods. You may also be able to find online nutrient listings for the foods served at fast-food and sit-down restaurant chains by typing the name of the chain into a search engine. Many fast-food restaurants also have printed nutrient listings available in-store for customers.

There are also many printed nutrient guides available for purchase online and in bookstores. (Be sure the one you choose lists the nutrient information you need.) Among them is one I compiled that combines nutrient listings (including fiber) for more than 2,500 foods, with additional details on carb counting. It's called *The Ultimate Guide to Accurate Carb Counting,* and it is available through Integrated Diabetes Services (877–735–3648 or www.integrateddiabetes.com).

than the listed serving size, you need to adjust the carbohydrate total accordingly. In the example above, the serving size is $\frac{1}{2}$ cup. If you consume a full cup, which is twice the amount of a single serving, you need to double the 26 grams of digestible carbs, for a grand total of 52 grams to include in your carb count.

3. Portion Conversion

This highly practical (but not as precise) technique for counting carbs makes use of portion estimation and is particularly useful when you're having a complex meal, dining out, or enjoying foods that vary in size. *Portion estimation* involves using a common object such as your fist, a tennis ball, or a milk carton to estimate the volume of a food. Once you've estimated the volume of your portion in this way, you then convert the volume measurement into a carb count based on the typical amount of carbohydrate per unit volume for that type of food.

A Handy Measure

When using portion conversion to count carbs, the fist of an average adult is considered equal to one cup. To find out if your own fist is roughly equal to one cup, take a large measuring cup or bowl and fill it halfway with water. Then immerse your fist completely in the water, and see how much the water level rises.

Confused yet? Don't be. Here's an example that should make this very clear: If you know that one cup of fruit juice contains about

30 grams of carbohydrate, and you are having a portion of juice equal to 1½ cups, you are having 30 × 1.5, or 45, grams of carbohydrate.

The key to making this method work is to obtain a fairly accurate size estimate for your food portion. Below are some common "measuring devices" that can be used for physically "seeing" or mentally "visualizing" portion volumes:

Adult's palm = approx. 4" diameter

Adult's spread hand = approx. 8" diameter

Average adult's fist = approx. 1 cup

Child's fist = approx. ½ cup

Cupped hand = approx. ½ cup

Deck of cards = approx. ⅓ cup

Half-pint milk = 1 cup

Large handful = approx. 1 cup

Soda can (12 oz.) = 1½ cups

Tennis ball = approx. ¾ cup

Keep in mind that *volume* consists of three dimensions: length, width, *and* height. The thickness or "tallness" of the food item should be taken into account when estimating the volume. Also, be sure to count only the portion that you are actually going to eat. The rind or peel on fruit, for example, should not be counted, nor should potato skins or bread crusts if you don't plan to eat them.

Below are approximate carb counts for standard portion sizes:

Bread, dense (bagel/soft pretzel) = 50g/cup

Bread/long sandwich roll = 8g/inch

Cake/muffin/pie = 50g/cup

Cereal, cold = 25g/cup

Chips = 15g/cup

Cookie = 20g/4" diameter

Fruit, summer = 20g/cup

Fruit, winter = 25g/cup

Ice cream = 35g/cup

Juice = 30g/cup

Milk = 12g/cup

Pancake, thin = 8g/4" diameter

Pasta, plain = 35g/cup

Pizza = 40g/8" diameter

Popcorn = 5g/cup

Potato = 30g/cup

Pretzels = 25g/cup

Rice, "sticky" = 75g/cup

Rice, instant = 50g/cup

Rolls = 25g/cup

Salad = 5g/cup

Soda, nondiet = 30g/cup

Sports drink = 15g/cup

Tortilla = 15g/8" diameter

Vegetables, cooked = 10g/cup

Vegetables, raw = 5g/cup

Here's how you would make portion conversion work: According to the list above, the fist of an average-size adult is roughly equal to a one-cup portion. If a cup of instant rice contains 50 grams of carbohydrate and you eat 1½ fist-size portions of instant rice, you are consuming about 75 grams of carbohydrate. If you eat three large handfuls of chips, you are consuming about three cups worth, and since one cup of chips contains 15 grams of carbohydrate, your three cups (or large handfuls) of chips are supplying you with about 45 grams of carbs.

The best way to fine-tune your portion estimation skills is through practice. Estimate the volume of a food item (using your fist or another item of known volume for comparison), and then either look up the exact volume on the food's label or place it in a measuring cup. Doing this repeatedly will train your eye and your mind to estimate portions accurately.

4. Carb Factors

Using **carb factors** involves weighing a portion of food on a scale and then multiplying the weight of the food (in grams) by its carb factor (which represents the *percentage* of the food's weight that is carbohydrate). Doing so will produce a fairly precise carb count for that portion of food. For example, apples have a carb factor of .13, which means that 13 percent of an average apple's weight is carbohydrate. If an apple without its core weighs 120 grams, the carb content is 120 × .13, or 15.6, grams.

Carb factors should only take into account the food that will actually be eaten. Foods should be weighed *without* the core, peel, rind, skin, seeds, packaging, crust, or any other part that will not actually be consumed.)

Carb factors are most helpful with foods eaten at home (nobody expects you to carry a scale everywhere you go), where the food may be an odd shape, the food density can vary considerably, or the food is actually a mixture of several foods. Examples include beef stew, homemade breads/pastries, and baked potatoes.

To figure the carb factor for packaged food, divide the total grams of carbohydrate in a serving (see label) by the weight of a serving. For example, if a serving of pastry contains 60 grams of carb and weighs 150 grams, its carb factor is 60 ÷ 150, or .40. You could then weigh any size portion of that pastry and multiply by .40 to determine the exact carb count.

GLYCEMIC INDEX

Now that you understand carb counting, it's time for a revelation: Not all carbs are created equal. While virtually all of the digestible carbs you consume will eventually be converted by your body into blood glucose, some make the transition much faster than others. The rate at which different carbs are converted into blood glucose can be compared using something called the **Glycemic Index (GI)**. A food's GI score, therefore, is another factor to take into account when considering the effect a food will have on blood sugar.

The GI ranks foods on a scale from 0 to 100. At the top, with a score of 100, is pure glucose (listed as dextrose on package labels). Other foods are ranked in comparison to the absorption rate of pure glucose. (There's a list of GI scores for many common foods at the end of the book.)

What the score actually represents is the percentage of a food's carbohydrate content that turns into blood glucose within the two hours after the food is eaten. Foods with a high GI score (above 70) tend to be digested and converted into glucose the fastest, producing a significant peak in blood sugar 30 to 45 minutes after they are eaten. Foods with a moderate GI score of 45 to 70 digest a bit slower, resulting in a less pronounced peak in blood sugar approximately one to two hours after they are eaten. Foods with a low GI score (below 45) have a slow, gradual effect on the blood sugar level: The peak is usually quite modest and may take several hours to occur.

White bread, for example, has a GI score of 71, and an apple has a score of 38. Their respective scores tell you that the white bread will raise blood sugar much faster than the apple will. Interestingly, wheat bread, with a score of 68, raises blood sugar almost as quickly as white bread does. On the other hand, sweet potatoes, with a score of 44, are much slower to raise blood sugar than are baked white potatoes, which have a score of 85. So it's not always easy to correctly guess a food's score.

Still, most starchy foods have a relatively high GI score: They are easily digested and quickly converted into blood sugar. Exceptions include starches found in legumes (dried beans and peas) and pasta. Foods that contain dextrose tend to rank very high on the Index. Fructose (fruit sugar) and lactose (milk sugar) are converted into blood sugar more slowly than are most starches.

Glycemic Index Rules of Thumb

- High-fiber foods raise blood sugar more slowly than low-fiber foods do.
- High-fat foods raise blood sugar more slowly than low-fat foods do.
- Solids raise blood sugar more slowly than liquids do.
- Cold foods raise blood sugar more slowly than hot foods do.
- Unripe foods raise blood sugar more slowly than ripe foods do.
- Raw foods raise blood sugar more slowly than cooked foods do.

Table sugar (sucrose) has a moderate GI score because it contains a combination of quickly converted glucose and more slowly converted fructose. Foods that contain fiber or large amounts of fat tend to have lower GI scores than do low-fat foods and foods without fiber.

Why care about GI scores? Because the effect that different foods have on your blood sugar is what really matters. In general, consuming primarily low-GI foods tends to make blood sugar easier to control. These foods enhance the feeling of fullness and help curb appetite. In a person who is insulin resistant or whose pancreas has difficulty making large amounts of insulin all at once, low-GI foods are better tolerated. When low-GI foods are eaten, the pancreas is able to control blood sugar by releasing insulin gradually; it doesn't have to produce a huge burst of insulin to keep up with a sudden flood of sugar into the bloodstream. Eating a diet of slowly digesting (low-GI) foods simply works better for people with diabetes because it eases the workload on the pancreas, prevents post-meal "spikes" in blood sugar, and provides a satisfying form of slow-burning fuel.

Below are some commonsense substitutions you can try:

MEAL	HIGH-GI CHOICES	LOWER-GI CHOICES
Breakfast	Typical cold cereal, bagel, toast, waffle, pancake, corn muffin	High-fiber cereal, oatmeal, yogurt, whole fruit, milk, bran muffin
Lunch	Sandwich made with white or whole-wheat bread, French fries, tortillas, canned pasta	Chili, pumpernickel bread, corn, carrots, raw salad vegetables
Dinner	Rice, rolls, white potato, canned vegetables	Sweet potato, pasta, beans, fresh or steamed vegetables
Snacks	Pretzels, chips, crackers, cake, donut	Popcorn, whole fruit, frozen yogurt

Calories & Weight Loss

Calories are really just energy for your body, the way gasoline is energy for a car. If you fill the gas tank, the car has plenty of energy to go where you need it to go. If you overfill the tank, the extra gas has to go somewhere; usually it spills all over and creates a fire hazard.

Likewise, if you consume more calories than your body uses for fuel, the extra calories have to go somewhere. Typically, they get stored as fat. That fat can only be eliminated if you start to burn more calories than you take in. It doesn't matter where the calories come from, whether it's carbohydrate, protein, fat, or alcohol. Plain and simple, if you eat more than you burn, you gain weight, and if you burn more than you eat, you lose weight.

The reason people with diabetes must pay such careful attention to calorie intake is that body fat interferes with insulin's action, causing or exacerbating insulin resistance. Each person's daily calorie needs are unique and are based on factors such as height, current weight, ideal weight, metabolism, and physical activity level. As was the case in determining appropriate carbohydrate intake, it is best to seek the guidance of a registered dietitian to help you figure out how many calories you should aim to consume each day.

Counting calories can be done similarly to counting carbs: You can check the label on packaged foods for calorie content per serving, and you can look up the calorie content of unlabeled foods either on the government's free online nutrient database or in a store-bought nutrient guide.

> ## Add to Subtract
>
> In weight loss terms, you're said to have "hit a plateau" when you've reached a certain weight and can't seem to lose any more pounds. When this happens, sometimes the cure is to take in *more* rather than fewer calories. How could that be? If you take in too few calories, your metabolism (the rate at which your body burns calories to fuel its processes and activities) may actually slow down. The body thinks it is starving and lowers its metabolic rate to conserve what few calories are coming in. So if you've hit a plateau, try taking in a few more calories each day to see if your metabolic rate resets and you begin losing pounds again.

If you want to maintain your current weight, find the approximate number of calories you should take in each day in the chart on the next page and use it as a rough starting point. If your goal, on the other hand, is to lose excess pounds of body fat, you will need to consume fewer calories each day than the amount listed in the chart.

DAILY CALORIES NEEDED TO MAINTAIN CURRENT WEIGHT

	Short Stature		Medium Stature		Tall Stature	
	Male	Female	Male	Female	Male	Female
Fairly Inactive	1,600	1,400	2,000	1,700	2,300	2,000
Moderately Active	2,100	1,900	2,600	2,200	3,100	2,600
Very Active	2,300	2,100	2,900	2,500	3,400	2,900

To lose excess body fat, you must burn more calories than you take in. Increasing your physical activity will help to create a calorie deficit. But exercise alone, with no change in caloric intake, rarely results in significant, sustainable weight loss. Most often, a combination of increased calorie expenditure and a modestly reduced calorie intake leads to the greatest weight loss over the long-term.

To meet the reasonable goal of losing one pound of fat per week, you will need to create a 3,500-calorie deficit each week. Adding 30 minutes of exercise most days will get you about halfway there. To make it the rest of the way, you will need to reduce your calorie intake. Cutting just 250 to 300 calories from your daily intake should get the job done.

If adding up the calories in everything you eat doesn't sound practical, don't worry. You can certainly cut your calorie intake just by paying more attention to your diet and using the commonsense techniques that follow. In fact, the reason most commercial diets produce weight loss is simply that they force dieters to think about and plan their daily food intake instead of just eating whatever they feel like eating!

TRUSTED CALORIE-CUTTING TECHNIQUES

What follows are 15 bonafide ways to make calorie cutting easier and more successful.

1. Publicize your intentions.

Writing down your goals and putting them on prominent display on your refrigerator or bathroom mirror will help refresh your commitment every day. Share your goals with family, friends, and co-workers, since the more people who know your intentions, the more support and encouragement you'll receive. And make those goals specific and realistic: "Lose lots of weight" and "eat less" are not specific. "Cut 300 calories a day" or "stop snacking after dinner" are realistic and specific goals.

2. Make sure your blood sugar is well-controlled.

Uncontrolled blood sugar levels make it difficult to control food intake. High blood sugar levels tend to increase appetite, and low blood sugar requires treatment with extra calories.

I know what you're thinking: "How can I control my blood sugar if I don't yet have my eating under control?" You may need to begin, increase, or add diabetes medication to get your blood sugar into a range that will allow you to get your eating under control. Then in time, as your weight comes down, you will probably be able to cut back on the medication.

Likewise, if your current medication program is causing hypo-glycemia more than once or twice a week, talk with your doctor about reducing your dose or switching to a different drug. Hypo-glycemia requires immediate calorie intake in the form of rapid-acting carbs and often causes a nearly insatiable appetite, so eliminating the lows can erase the need for those hundreds of extra calories each week.

3. Write it all down.

Most people underestimate their food intake by 20 percent or more. Starting a food diary will help you become more aware of what you're actually eating. Start with a blank notebook and, for two weeks, write down precisely what, when, and how much you take in (down to a stick of gum). Be honest and specific (a "baked potato" is not the same as a "baked potato with sour cream, cheddar, and bacon bits"). To make your diary even more effective, also record the *context:* where you were, what you were doing, and how you were feeling when you ate. Such details can reveal patterns and provide insight into your eating habits. After two weeks, review your diary to see what your usual food intake and eating habits are really like. Then gradually implement the strategies and tips discussed here, keeping records as you go. Once you've attained your goal weight, continue filling in your diary; it will help you maintain your weight loss long term.

4. Don't skip meals.

It is better to eat three meals a day than just two. Having three substantial, evenly spaced meals at roughly the same times each day helps the body to regulate its appetite according to your schedule. Skipping meals tends to cause cravings and intense hunger late in the day, which usually leads to uncontrolled snacking and poor food choices. Indeed, research has shown that people who skip meals tend to take in more calories through the course of the day than those who don't skip meals.

5. Reduce your fat intake.

Fat is much more calorie dense than carbohydrate, protein, or even alcohol. Every gram of fat contains nine calories, whereas a gram of alcohol contains seven and a gram of carbohydrate or protein contains just four. By choosing a low-fat food in place of a high-fat food of equal size, you are likely to eliminate many calories. For example, a four-ounce serving of low-fat frozen yogurt contains about 100 calories, while four ounces of ice cream contain about 150. Although the portions are the same, one has more carbohydrate, the other more fat. Just don't get the idea that something will help you lose weight just because it is low in fat. If it contains carbohydrate, protein, or alcohol, it still has calories, and it can still cause weight gain if eaten in large quantities. (Some low-fat versions even contain *more* calories than their full-fat counterparts, so check labels carefully!)

To help trim fat from your diet:

- Select low-fat snacks. Instead of chips, nuts, cookies, and chocolate, choose low-fat popcorn, low-fat or nonfat yogurt, or fresh fruits and vegetables.

- Eat out less. Food prepared at a restaurant, whether that's a quality sit-down establishment, a fast-food outlet, or a take-out joint, tends to contain a great deal more fat than food that is prepared at home.

- Switch to skim milk. Whole and even two-percent milk contain a great deal more fat. Opt for reduced-fat varieties of other dairy products, as well.

- Choose lean cuts of meat. The more "marbling" throughout a cut of beef, the more fat it contains. White-meat poultry and seafood tend to be lower in fat than fowl, dark-meat poultry, beef, and pork. Also, remove the skin prior to eating fowl or poultry.

6. Vegify your plate.

Consider how much space different foods take up on your plate. The traditional meal contains a main course of meat, a substantial side of something starchy, and a small portion of vegetable, creating a plate that is divided something like this:

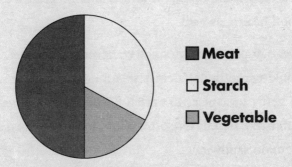

But meat tends to be high in calories, and starch tends to drive up blood sugar. Vegetables, on the other hand, are typically low in calories and have low GI scores. So give vegetables the place of honor, and take a smaller portion of meat and a much smaller portion of starch, for a plate that looks more like this:

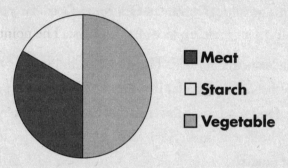

Making leafy and crunchy vegetables (fresh or cooked) a more substantial part of every meal helps increase the fiber content of your diet. Because most vegetables are low on the GI chart, they provide slow-burning fuel. They have "volume," so they tend to fill you up and curb your appetite, making it easier to skip second helpings. Vegetables are rich in vitamins and minerals we all need for good health, as well.

Get creative. Sample vegetables you've never tried before. Try different cooking methods, such as steaming, grilling, or stir-frying. Use herbs and spices to enrich flavors. Use seasonal vegetables to make frittatas, risotto, pilafs, or clear soups, or try layering them on sandwiches.

7. Pay attention to portion sizes.

One of my brightest patients, a college professor, couldn't figure out why his weight kept going up. When I asked him to describe his breakfast, he said, "All I'm having is a cup of cereal, half a cup of milk, and a piece of toast." When I had him actually *measure* his breakfast, he found he was really having almost two cups of cereal, a full cup of milk, and extra-thick toast. The point? Even if you make healthy food choices, you can undermine your weight-loss efforts with oversize portions. Invest in a set of measuring cups and spoons and a basic food scale, and test your ability to "eyeball" portions from time to time.

The typical portion size of many foods has increased dramatically over the past several decades. Today's 20-ounce soda used to be only 8 ounces. The 30-gram bagel has been supplanted by a monstrous 70-gram one. Even movie-theater popcorn has busted its own beltline: A "large" popcorn from the '60s is smaller than a "small" popcorn at most theaters today.

Reducing portion sizes across-the-board has worked for many dieters. Try eating 25 percent or 50 percent less of everything than you're used to having—main courses, side dishes, desserts, beverages. Simply *paying attention* to your portion sizes may be all it takes to cut down significantly on your calorie intake!

One trick that helps some people to eat less is to use smaller plates and bowls for serving meals. A portion of food that is served on a small plate seems larger than the same portion presented on a large plate.

Restaurants are notorious for serving huge portions. So when you eat out, consider ordering child-size portions or asking that half your serving be placed in a doggie bag before it reaches your table. And steer clear of "all you can eat" buffets!

8. Take your time.

It can take 30 to 60 minutes for the "full" sensation to register, even after a substantial meal. So slow down. Chew each mouthful thoroughly, and put your fork down between bites. And after finishing your usual portion, get up from the table and do something else: Clear and clean the dishes, take a walk, read your mail, etc. By the time you're done, the feeling of fullness should be setting in, and you will have kept yourself from eating more than you need.

Small and Frequent Wins the Race

For people who have type 2 diabetes, eating several small meals per day actually tends to produce better blood sugar control than having just three large meals. The only exceptions are the people who take insulin at each meal. For them, giving the insulin time to finish working before eating again produces the best blood sugar control, so they tend to do better with just the three large meals.

9. Try nixing snacks.

If you eat three substantial meals, consider eliminating snacks. If you eat smaller meals that are more than four hours apart, it is reasonable to have a modest snack between those meals. If you do snack, though, be sure to measure out what you are going to eat; don't eat directly from a full-size bag, package, or container.

10. Drink plenty of water.

The recommended water intake per day is about two quarts (eight cups). Research has even shown that your basal metabolic rate (the amount of calories your body burns at rest) may increase up to 30 percent when you start drinking enough water. Thirst is also often mistaken for hunger, so before you snack, drink a glass of water first to see if the feeling of hunger passes. If you don't like plain water, try adding a twist of lemon or lime or a *small* splash of juice. Decaffeinated tea and coffee, calorie-free drinks, and seltzer also count toward your eight cups a day.

11. Avoid "cheap" calories.

It's amazing how many calories we take in without realizing it. Sugary beverages are a good example. A single can of regular soda contains 130 to 180 calories; a can of diet soda usually contains none. Choose sugar-free beverages instead.

Sauces, dressings, and gravies are another source of cheap calories. A healthy 100-calorie salad can easily become a 400- to

500-calorie monster when doused in Caesar dressing. Use toppings in moderation, and skip cream-based varieties.

12. Cut down on alcohol.

Like fat, alcohol is very dense in calories. Alcohol contains seven calories per gram, and that's not counting the calories from the carbohydrates that accompany the alcohol in beer, wine, and mixed drinks. Alcohol consumption also interferes with the body's burning of excess fat for fuel. Because alcohol is a toxin the body wants to get rid of as quickly as possible, the body holds off using stored fat for fuel and instead burns the alcohol for fuel. So if you're serious about losing weight and gaining control of your blood sugar, opt for seltzer or diet soda rather than alcoholic beverages most or all of the time.

13. Prepare to be hungry sometimes.

There will be times when you'll want to eat when you shouldn't. Remember, however, that you *are* stronger and smarter than your appetite. These strategies may help you handle cravings:

- Since many food cravings are situational rather than physical, try slowly counting to 30 when a craving strikes. It will usually subside.

- When a craving hits, visualize yourself thinner and more fit. Then decide which will make you feel better: looking and feeling that way or eating the food you're craving.

- Engage in a (healthy or neutral) substitute habit when a craving occurs: Make and drink tea, chew sugarless gum, take a short walk, text a friend, meditate, etc.

- If you tend to get cravings in certain situations, change your routine. Do something other than watching TV in the evening. Stay out of the kitchen unless you're preparing or eating a meal. Don't allow food in the car.

14. Rule out—or treat—other health problems.

Controlling your eating patterns is not always easy. The last thing you need is a secondary health condition that interferes with your efforts.

Compulsive eating disorders, for example, occur in nearly half of all overweight people. Binge eating may have a physical or psychological basis that can be treated with therapy and/or medication. Symptoms include:

- Eating large quantities of high-calorie foods
- Eating secretively
- Frequent weight fluctuations of more than ten pounds
- Feeling depressed after eating
- Feeling that you cannot control your eating

Without realizing it, many people use food for comfort or distraction. Some people are psychologically addicted to food, and they use it as a way of self-medicating an underlying psychological problem. If you habitually use food to make yourself feel better, talk to a therapist who specializes in eating disorders.

Depression is another medical disorder common among people with diabetes. Depression can lead to unhealthy eating patterns. Symptoms include:

- Frequent feelings of sadness or dread of the future

- Crying spells

- Fatigue

- Dwelling on negative thoughts

- Suicidal thoughts (If you experience these, seek immediate medical attention.)

Talk to your doctor if you experience these or similar symptoms. Talk/behavioral therapy and/or medication can be used quite successfully to treat depression.

Hypothyroidism ("underactive thyroid") is very common among people who have had diabetes for many years. Thyroid hormone plays a major role in regulating metabolism, so hypothyroidism can make weight loss very difficult. Symptoms of hypothyroidism include:

- Feeling sluggish

- Decreased appetite

- Slowed reflexes

- Weight gain

- Constipation

- Inability to tolerate cold

Medications for treating hypothyroidism can reverse these symptoms and help restore metabolism to a normal level.

If you suspect that you may have a secondary health condition that is interfering with your ability to lose excess body fat, consult your doctor.

15. Discuss medication with your doctor.

A number of diabetes medications have been shown to also curb hunger and help people with type 2 to eat less. Metformin reduces the amount of sugar released by the liver, but it can also cause mild stomach upset and loss of appetite. The injectable drug Byetta (exenatide) improves the ability of the pancreas to produce insulin and slows the rate at which food moves from the stomach into the intestines, which triggers a strong feeling of fullness soon after you start eating. Symlin (pramlintide), another injectable that slows stomach emptying, also stimulates the satiety (fullness) center of the brain, helping to reduce food cravings. Consider asking your doctor if any of these medications is appropriate for you.

STEP 11:
Call in the Cavalry

If you can't maintain good control with lifestyle tools alone, it's time to add medication to your arsenal.

L ET THERE BE no doubt: A healthy lifestyle is the best and most effective way to manage blood sugar levels if you have or are at risk for type 2 diabetes. But sometimes, a healthy lifestyle by itself is not enough to get the whole job done. Sometimes, medication is required. Fortunately, the drugs available today to treat diabetes are safer, easier to take, and more effective than ever before.

Diabetes medication may be needed under two conditions:

1. You have been doing the right things from a lifestyle standpoint for at least three months, but your blood sugar level is still above your target range.

2. Elevated blood sugar is keeping you from wielding your lifestyle tools. The short-term effects of high blood sugar, including increased appetite and lack of energy, are not exactly conducive to eating properly and being physically active. And continuing to see those high readings, despite your efforts, can cause considerable stress.

It's important to note that needing medication is not a sign of failure. It's a simple fact of life when you suffer from a progressive disease such as diabetes. Even if you make all the recommended lifestyle adjustments, there's still a decent chance that, at some point, your lifestyle tools will no longer be enough to control your blood sugar, and you will need medication. The only failure would be if you found yourself in either of the situations noted above and didn't take advantage of the diabetes medications available.

So if lifestyle changes aren't doing the job for you, work with your doctor to understand the medication options—pills, injectables, and insulin—and determine which is/are most appropriate at the current stage of your condition. Talk to your other team members to find out what changes you might need to make in your diet or physical activity as a result of adding medication (because you *must* continue using your lifestyle tools even after you begin using medication). Be sure you know how and when to administer your medication. And, most important of all, be sure to take the medication properly and without fail, because that is the only way it will help save you from the ravages of out-of-control blood sugar.

APPENDIX A:
Strength-Training Exercises

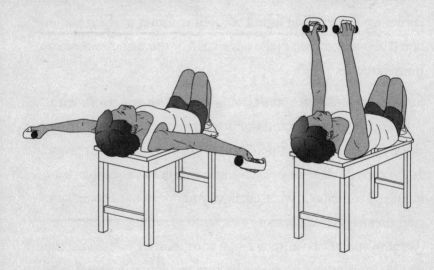

Chest Fly

1. Lie flat on bench (or floor), a weight in each hand, arms extended straight out to the sides with elbows loose, knees bent, and feet flat on bench.

2. Keeping arms extended and lower back against bench at all times, slowly raise arms up above chest.

3. Slowly lower arms to starting position to complete one rep.

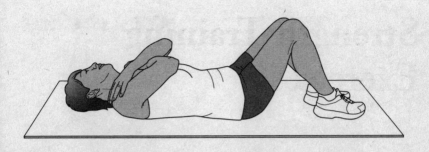

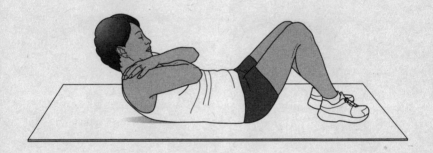

Abdominal Crunch

1. Lie on mat, arms crossed loosely over upper chest, knees bent, and feet flat on mat.

2. Slowly raise head and lift shoulders slightly off mat.

3. Slowly lower head and shoulders back down to mat to complete one rep.

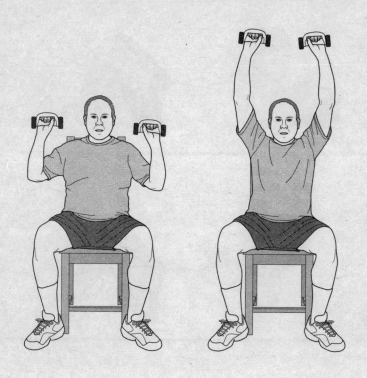

Shoulder Press

1. Sit with back against chair back, a weight in each hand held just above shoulder height, palms facing forward, and feet flat on floor.

2. Keeping back against chair back and palms facing forward, raise weights directly overhead.

3. Slowly lower weights to starting position to complete one rep.

174

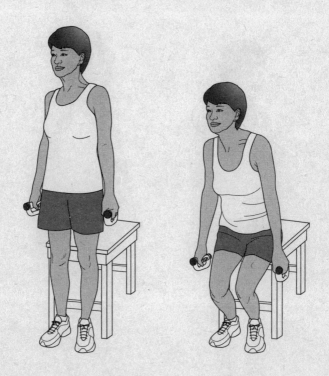

Squat to Bench

1. Stand just in front of chair or bench, with arms down at sides and a weight in each hand.

2. Keeping back straight, slowly bend knees until buttocks just touch seat, but do not sit down.

3. Slowly straighten knees and return to starting position to complete one rep.

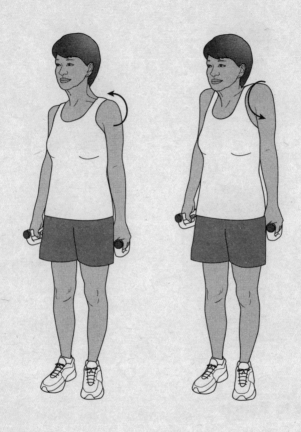

Shrug

1. Stand with arms down at sides, a weight in each hand.

2. Slowly roll shoulders in circular motion, first backwards, then upwards, then frontwards, then back down to starting position to complete one rep.

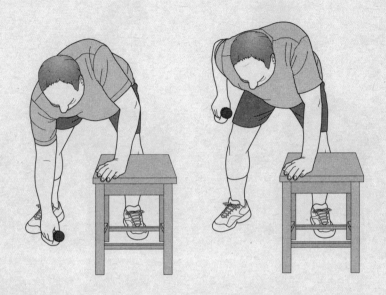

Upward Row

1. Bend forward at hips, placing one hand on bench or chair seat for support. Hold weight in other hand, allowing arm to dangle straight down.

2. Slowly lift weight—keeping arm close to body—until elbow reaches height of torso.

3. Slowly lower weight to starting position to complete one rep. After completing one set, repeat with opposite arm.

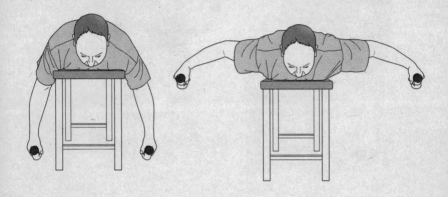

Inverted Fly

1. Lie facedown on bench, neck aligned with spine, arms dangling down on either side of bench, a weight in each hand.

2. Slowly raise arms outward, keeping them straight as possible without locking elbows, until they reach height of torso.

3. Slowly lower weights to starting position to complete one rep.

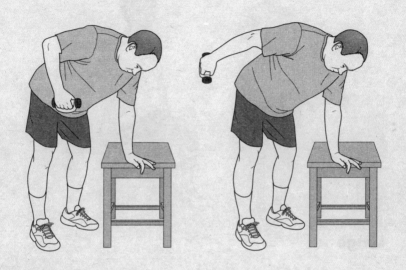

Triceps Extension

1. Bend forward at hips, placing one hand on bench for support. Hold weight in other hand, and, keeping upper arm close to side and parallel to torso, bend arm so elbow forms right angle and weight dangles straight down.

2. Slowly straighten elbow, extending weight backward to height of torso.

3. Slowly bend elbow and lower weight to starting position to complete one rep. After one set, repeat with other arm.

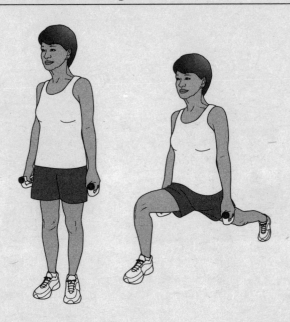

Lunge

1. Stand straight, feet comfortably apart, arms down at sides, a weight in each hand.

2. Keeping back perpendicular to floor and toes pointing forward throughout exercise, take giant step forward with right leg. Slowly lower torso by bending right knee until it is aligned directly above (not beyond) right ankle, with right thigh parallel to floor and lower leg perpendicular to it. Keep left leg extended backward, toes on floor.

3. Slowly straighten right leg and raise torso, then step back with right leg to return to starting position. Repeat using left leg to step forward, and return to starting position to complete one rep.

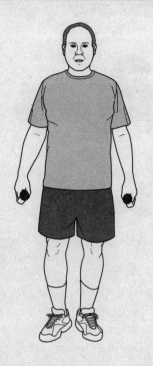 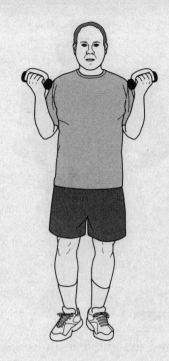

Arm Curl

1. Stand straight, feet comfortably apart, arms at sides, a weight in each hand.

2. Slowly bend elbows and raise weights to shoulder height. As you raise weights in front of your body, turn your lower arms slightly so your inner wrists face upward during lift.

3. Slowly lower weights back to starting position to complete one rep.

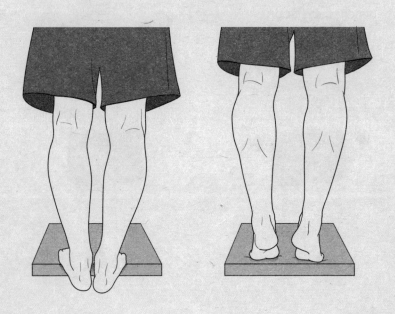

Heel Raise

1. Stand with feet on end of thick mat or board or bottom stair, heels hanging down off edge. Place hand against railing or nearby sturdy object for balance, if necessary.

2. Use lower leg muscles to slowly raise heels up above surface.

3. Slowly lower heels back down to starting position to complete one rep.

Forearm Wrist Curl

A1. Sit on edge of bench, feet flat on floor, forearms resting on thighs, inner wrists facing upward, and a weight in each hand. Let hands hang down, unsupported by thighs.

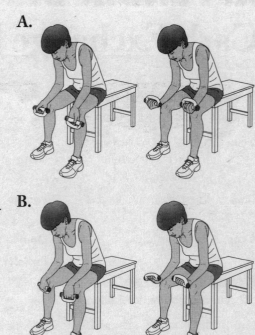

A2. Curl weights up without lifting forearms from thighs.

A3. Lower weights to starting position to complete one rep.

B1. After completing one set with inner wrists facing upward, turn hands over, so inner wrists face downward. Rest forearms on thighs, and let hands hang down, unsupported by thighs.

B2. Curl weights up without lifting forearms from thighs.

B3. Lower weights to starting position to complete one rep.

183

APPENDIX B:
Carb Exchange List

1 Vegetable Exchange
(5 grams carbohydrate) equals:

½ cup	Vegetables, cooked (carrots, broccoli, zucchini, cabbage, etc.)
1 cup	Vegetables, raw, or salad greens
½ cup	Vegetable juice

1 Milk Exchange
(12 grams carbohydrate) equals:

1 cup	Milk: fat-free, 1% fat, 2%, or whole
¾ cup	Yogurt, plain nonfat or low-fat
1 cup	Yogurt, artificially sweetened

1 Meat Exchange
(0 grams carbohydrate) equals:

1 ounce	Beef, pork, turkey, or chicken
1 ounce	Fish fillet (flounder, sole, scrod, cod, etc.)
1 ounce	Tuna or sardines, canned
1 ounce	Shellfish (clams, lobster, scallops, shrimp)
¾ cup	Cottage cheese, nonfat or low-fat
1 ounce	Cheese, shredded or sliced
1 ounce	Lunch meat
1 whole	Egg
¼ cup	Egg substitute
4 ounces	Tofu

1 Fruit Exchange
(15 grams carbohydrate) equals:

1 small	Apple, banana, orange, or nectarine
1 medium	Peach
1	Kiwi
½	Grapefruit or mango
1 cup	Berries, fresh (strawberries, raspberries, blueberries)
1 cup	Melon, fresh, cubes

1 slice	Melon, honeydew or cantaloupe
½ cup	Juice (orange, apple, or grape)
4 teaspoons	Jelly or jam

1 Starch Exchange
(15 grams carbohydrate) equals:

1 slice	Bread (white, pumpernickel, whole-wheat, rye)
2 slices	Bread, reduced-calorie or "lite"
¼ (1 ounce)	Bagel, bakery-style
½	Bagel, frozen, or English muffin
½	Bun, hamburger or hot dog
1 small	Dinner roll
¾ cup	Cold cereal
⅓ cup	Rice (cooked), brown or white
⅓ cup	Barley or couscous, cooked
⅓ cup	Legumes (dried beans, peas, lentils)
½ cup	Beans, cooked (black or kidney beans, chick peas)
½ cup	Pasta, cooked

½ cup	Corn, potato, or green peas
3 ounces	Potato, baked, sweet or white
¾ ounce	Pretzels
3 cups	Popcorn, air-popped or microwaved

1 Fat Exchange
(0 grams carbohydrate) equals:

1 teaspoon	Oil (vegetable, corn, canola, olive, etc.)
1 teaspoon	Butter
1 teaspoon	Margarine, stick
1 teaspoon	Mayonnaise
1 Tablespoon	Margarine or mayonnaise, reduced-fat
1 Tablespoon	Salad dressing
1 Tablespoon	Cream cheese
2 Tablespoons	Lite cream cheese
⅛	Avocado
8 large	Black olives
10 large	Green olives, stuffed
1 slice	Bacon

185

APPENDIX C:
Glycemic Index of Common Foods

BREAD/CRACKERS

Bagel	72
Graham crackers	74
Hamburger bun	61
Kaiser roll	73
Pita bread	57
Pumpernickel bread	51
Rye bread, dark	76
Rye bread, light	55
Saltines	74
Sourdough bread	52
Wheat bread, high-fiber	68
White bread	71

CAKES/COOKIES/MUFFINS

Angel food cake	67
Banana bread	47
Blueberry muffin	59
Chocolate cake	38
Corn muffin	102
Cupcake with icing	73
Donut	76
Oat bran muffin	60
Oatmeal cookie	55
Pound cake	54
Shortbread cookies	64

CANDY

Jelly beans	80
Lifesavers	70
M&M's, peanut	33
Milky Way Bar	44

CEREALS/BREAKFAST

All-Bran	42
Bran flakes	74
Cheerios	74
Cocoa Krispies	77
Corn flakes	83
Cream of wheat	70
Frosted Flakes	55
Golden Grahams	71
Grape Nuts	67
Life	66
Oatmeal	49
Pancakes	67
Puffed Wheat	67
Raisin Bran	73
Rice Bran	19
Rice Krispies	82
Shredded Wheat	69
Special K	66
Total	76
Waffles	76

DAIRY

Chocolate milk	34
Ice cream, vanilla	62
Ice cream, chocolate	68
Milk, skim	32
Milk, whole	27
Soy milk	30
Yogurt, low-fat	33

FRUITS/JUICES
Apple 38
Apple juice 41
Apricot 57
Banana 55
Cantaloupe 65
Cherries 22
Cranberry juice 68
Dates 103
Fruit cocktail 55
Grapefruit 25
Grapefruit juice 48
Grapes 46
Orange 44
Orange juice 52
Peach 42
Pear 37
Pineapple 66
Pineapple juice 46
Plum 39
Raisins 64
Watermelon 72

LEGUMES
Baked beans 48
Black beans 30
Black-eyed peas 42
Chick peas 33
Fava beans 79
Lentils, red 25
Lima beans 32
Peas, dried 22
Pinto beans 45
Red kidney beans 19

PASTA
Fettuccini 32
Gnocchi 68
Linguini 55
Macaroni 45
Macaroni & cheese 64

Ravioli w/meat 39
Spaghetti 41
Spaghetti, wheat 37

RICE/GRAIN
Brown rice 55
Couscous 65
Instant rice 87
Long-grain rice 56
Risotto 69
Vermicelli 58

SNACK FOODS
Corn chips 74
Granola bar 61
Peanuts 15
Popcorn 55
Potato chips 54
Pretzels 81
Rice cakes 77

SOUPS
Black bean 64
Lentil 44
Minestrone 39
Split pea 60
Tomato 38

SUGARS/SPREADS
Honey 58
Strawberry jam 51

VEGETABLES
French fries 75
Potato, baked 85
Potato, mashed 91
Carrots, boiled 49
Carrots, raw 16
Corn, sweet 55
Peas 48
Sweet potato 44

Index